THE

CLEAN

HOLIDAY

COOKBOOK

Over 500 Dairy-Free/Gluten Free/Paleo/Whole/Nut-Free/Sugar-Free/Soy-Free/Grain-Free Allergen-Friendly Recipes to keep you healthy this festive Period

By

Maryann Hill

INTRODUCTION

When I called my mom to inform her I decided to tackle my second round of Paleo Diet last December, she was... less than thrilled. While she knew I would be happy to make my family tasty dinners while I was home, she dreaded the idea of her annual holiday feast being interrupted by some unforgiving dietary restrictions.

For those still unfamiliar with the clean eating phenomenon, Paleo Diet is a clean eating program that eliminates alcohol, sugars, dairy, grains, and legumes from your diet—a.k.a. all of the fun, festive things normally consumed in excess during the holidays. That meant no eggnog, no cider, no tree-shaped cookies dripping in sugary frosting, or butter-drenched rolls at the dinner table.

While the idea of tackling the holiday season without a drop of mulled wine or a nibble of sugar cookie might send a shiver up your spine, I was drawn to the idea of avoiding the high amounts of sweets and booze I typically consume throughout the holidays, and starting the new year feeling completely fresh and healthy. (Note: I had completed a 60 Days Paleo diet successfully before, so I felt more confident about my ability to follow through. If you're trying your first round over the holidays, prepare to have your willpower seriously tested.)

The book contains over 500 recipes with nutritional information for all 7 basic allergies and diet which include but not limited to Dairy Free, Gluten Free, Paleo, Grain Free, Nut Free, Sugar Free, Soy Free, Whole 30 and even Recipe that can be tailored for AIP.

The scrumptious recipes are classified in Appetizers, Desserts, Breakfast, Main Dishes and Side Dishes, very easy to make and will help you lose weight while nourishing your body.

It has an Index to help you locate your Holiday meals during celebrations easily.

THE FIRST RULE OF THIS PALEO DIET

Is to not talk about it. The fact of the matter is that most people won't realize they're being deprived of any specific ingredients if it's not brought to their attention. Instead of mentioning the program constantly—after all, nobody really wants to hear about someone else's diet—serve up your Paleo dishes on the down low. Not only are family and guests unlikely to notice they're eating sugar-, grain- and dairy-free dishes, but they also won't be annoyed by your dietary reminders.

Make sure the wine and sugary treats are readily available for everyone else to imbibe in throughout your holiday celebrations. Although you won't be able to join in on the fun, your guests won't realize they're being served an otherwise Paleo-friendly feast if they have easy access to the rest of their festive favorites.

Main Dishes

One of the most convenient parts of sticking to your Whole foods program around the holidays is that protein recipes that please everyone, but won't break your dietary rules, are easy to come by. Many simple whole turkey recipes, like this Turkey Burgers with Kale, are Whole foods approved as long as you substitute ghee or coconut oil for standard butter. The Slow Cooker Turkey Breast and Roasted Turkey Breast with sweet potatoes will also go with Lemon, and Garlic

Or, give another bird a go with a Creamy Garlic Chicken (once again, swapping butter for ghee), or this completely Paleo-friendly Thai Chicken soup recipe, which also provides you with an excellent side dish.

If you're more of a fish fan, Grilled Salmon with Garlic, Lemon, and Basil is a perfect program-approved main that everyone at your table will love.

Salads

Salads are an easy way to combine tons of Paleo-friendly vegetables, nuts, oils, and vinegars for a satisfying and healthy starter to your meal. The Low Carb Cucumber salad will be a great base to work with, adding your own special ingredients and twists.

Sides

Many satisfying holiday sides can be easily made to fit within the confines of the program, and will be so filling and flavorful that no guest will suspect they're being deprived of any ingredients.

The simple roasted vegetable options are endless, like Roasted Potatoes, or try a more complex recipe like this Dijon Pomegranate roasted Brussel.

Recipes like Harvest Vegetable Hash and Garlic Mashed Potatoes are worth trying to.

Dessert

The dessert section of the meal will be your biggest holiday sacrifice—besides wine and eggnog, that is. Unfortunately, one of the basic rules of Whole foods diet is not attempting to recreate baked goods or junk food using approved ingredients, so trying to hunt down a vegan, sugar-free pumpkin pie recipe isn't exactly on the up-and-up.

While your family pigs out on apple pie a la mode, dense chocolate cakes, and all of the holiday cookies, make yourself some simple Confetti Turkey Burgers, and do your best not to longingly eye everyone else's slices of carrot cake.

Though it will be tough at the time, at the end of your feast—with both you and your family well fed and free of a single dietary regret—you'll able to sleep soundly with visions of sugarplums dancing in your head.

EXCERPTS

Oven Roasted Carrots

Thanksgiving | Christmas | New Year | Easter | Halloween

Prep Time: 5 minutes|| Cook Time: 25 minutes

Yield: 4

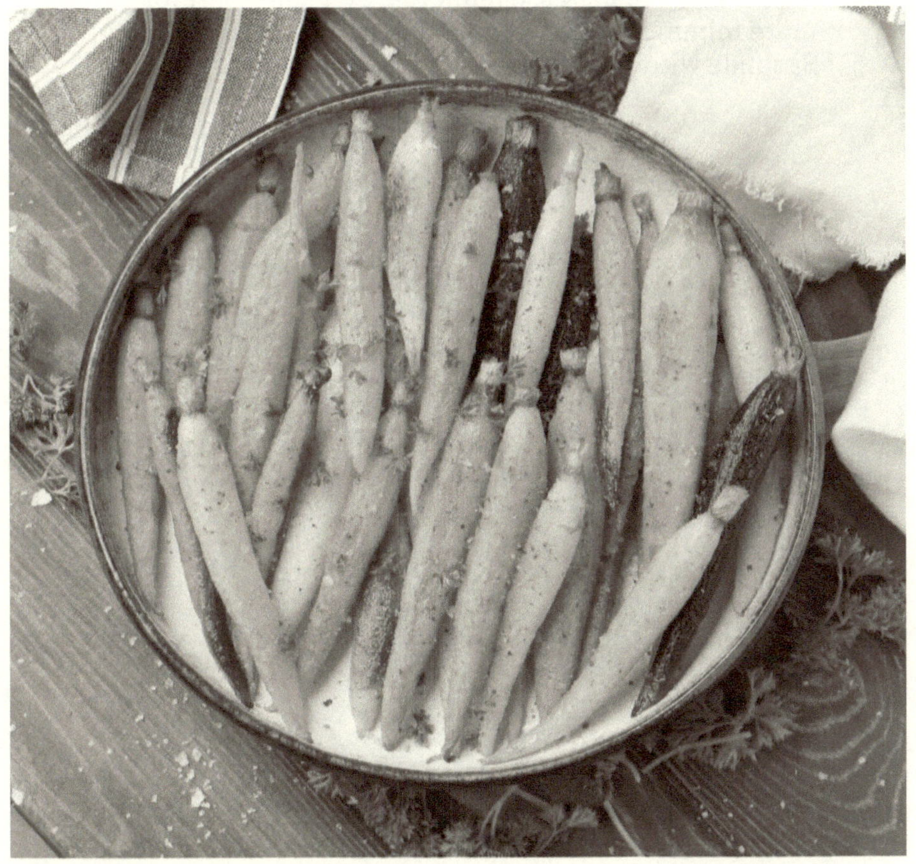

Save some time and make an easy holiday side dish. These Oven Roasted Carrots are a super simple side for your holiday menu or with a weeknight dinner. Rainbow carrots spiced with Adobo seasoning and roasted in the oven.

Ingredients

- 2 Lbs Rainbow Carrots, (trimmed, washed)
- 2 Tablespoons Olive Oil
- 1 teaspoon Adobo Seasoning

Instructions

1. Preheat oven to 400°F

2. Toss carrots with olive oil and seasoning. Transfer to a lightly oiled rimmed baking sheet.
3. Make sure the baking sheet is large enough that the carrots are spread out, otherwise use 2 baking sheets.
4. Roast carrots for 15 minutes.
5. Rotate carrots, increase temp to 425°F and roast for 10-15 more minutes or until tender and golden brown.
6. Sprinkle with salt, pepper, fresh parsley and serve.

Spicy Baked Shrimp with Cilantro Lime Dip

Prep Time: 5 minutes||Cook Time: 10 minutes

Thanksgiving | Christmas | New Year | Easter | Halloween

Yield: 4

Serving Size 1

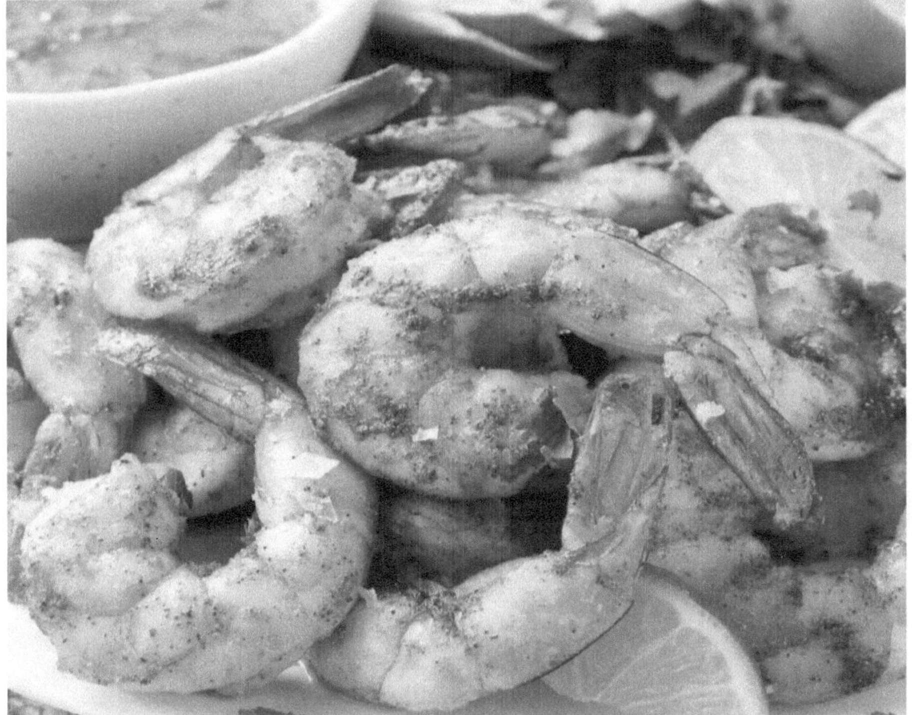

For punch in the face flavor, make these Cilantro Lime Spicy Baked Shrimp! This recipe starts with shrimp covered in spices, baked to perfection then served with a fresh cilantro lime dip.
Perfect for a healthy lunch, dinner, appetizer or a snack!

Ingredients

Spicy Shrimp
- 1 Lb . Large Wild Shrimp - thawed, peeled, deveined, tail-on
- 2 Tablespoons Olive Oil, (or avocado oil)
- 1/2 teaspoon Chili Powder

- 1/2 teaspoon Garlic Powder
- 1/4 teaspoon Cumin
- 1/4 teaspoon Onion Powder
- 1/4 teaspoon Sea Salt, or Kosher
- 1/8 teaspoon Ground Pepper

Cilantro Lime Dip
- Juice of 2 Small Limes
- Zest of 1 Lime
- 1/4 Cup Olive Oil, (or avocado oil)
- Handful Fresh Cilantro - stems removed, chopped
- Pinch Sea Salt

Instructions

Spicy Shrimp
1. Preheat oven to 400°F
2. Rinse and Drain thawed shrimp.
3. Toss shrimp with oil and spices. Transfer to a rimmed baking sheet.
4. Bake 8-10 minutes (depending on size) or until shrimp are pink and in a loose 'C' shape.

Cilantro Lime Dip
1. Whisk all ingredients for 1-2 minutes.
2. Serve with shrimp.

Calories 481, Total Fat 33g, Saturated Fat 5g, Trans Fat 0g, Unsaturated Fat 26g, Cholesterol 239mg, Sodium 1299mg, Carbohydrates 22g, Fiber 7g, Sugar 8g, Protein 28g

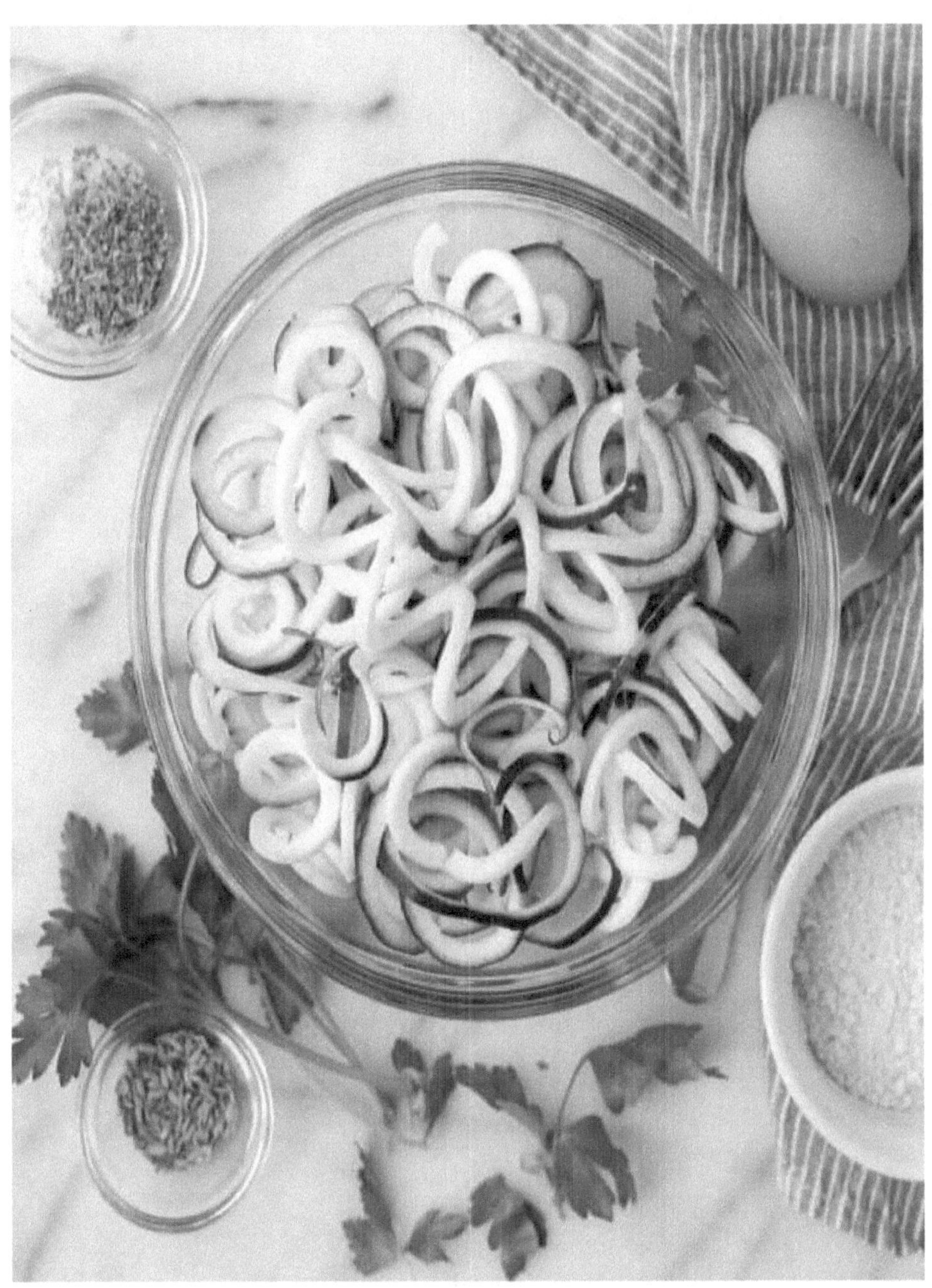

Meatballs and Sauce

Prep Time:25 mins||Cook Time:15 mins

Thanksgiving | Christmas | New Year | Easter | Halloween

Yield: 34 meatballs

Course: Main Course

Easy, DELICIOUS Italian Whole 30 meatballs and sauce with ground turkey, almond flour, and Italian seasoning. A healthy, low-carb recipe that families love!

Ingredients

FOR THE MEATBALLS:

- 1/4 cup blanched almond flour
- 1 1/2 teaspoons garlic powder
- 1 1/2 teaspoons dried oregano
- 1 teaspoon onion powder
- 1 teaspoon fennel seeds
- 1 teaspoon kosher salt
- 1/2 teaspoon crushed red pepper flakes — reduce to 1/4 teaspoon if sensitive to spice
- 1/4 teaspoon ground nutmeg
- 2 pounds 93% lean ground turkey
- 1 large egg — lightly beaten
- tablespoons finely chopped fresh parsley — plus additional for serving
- 24 ounces jarred prepared tomato-based pasta sauce* — or homemade pasta sauce, see below

For serving: Zucchini noodles — shredded spaghetti squash, or sweet potato noodles

IF YOU'D LIKE TO MAKE HOMEMADE WHOLE MARINARA SAUCE (see notes for store-bought options):

- 1 teaspoon extra-virgin olive oil
- 2 cloves garlic — minced
- 1 small onion — finely chopped
- 1/2 teaspoon kosher salt
- 1/4 teaspoon black pepper
- 1 can crushed tomatoes — (28 ounces)

* 1 can diced tomatoes (I like to use fire roasted for extra flavor) — (14 ounces)
* 1 teaspoon dried basil
* 1/2 teaspoon dried oregano

Instructions

1. Place two oven racks in the upper and lower thirds of the oven. Preheat the oven to 400 degrees F.
2. Line two baking sheets with aluminum foil and lightly coat them with nonstick spray, or line them with parchment paper or silicone baking mats. (If you are making vegetable noodles to serve with the meatballs, I recommend prepping them now so that they are ready to serve when the meatballs finish cooking.
3. If you are making homemade sauce, I like to start this simmering before the meatballs go in the oven so that it is ready as well.)
4. In a small bowl, whisk together the almond flour, garlic, oregano, onion powder, fennel, salt, red pepper flakes, and nutmeg until the ingredients are evenly combined.
5. Add the turkey to a large bowl. Sprinkle the almond flour mix over the top. Add the beaten egg and parsley. With a fork or your hands, gently combine the ingredients until everything is evenly distributed.
6. Be careful not to overwork or compact the meat, or the meatballs will be tough.
7. With a small scoop or spoon, scoop the meat and shape into 1 1/2-inch balls, again being careful not to compact the meat. Arrange on the baking sheets. You will have about 34 meatballs total. If using store-bought sauce, warm it up while the meatballs cook.
8. Bake for 10 minutes, and then remove the baking sheet from the oven. Using tongs, gently turn the meatballs and return them to the oven, switching the position of the sheet pans on the upper and lower racks. Continue baking until cooked through, about 5 additional minutes. Serve hot with vegetable noodles, sauce, and a sprinkle of fresh parsley.

For Homemade Whole 30 Tomato Pasta Sauce:

1. Heat the olive oil in a large, deep skillet over medium high. Add the garlic, onion, salt, and pepper.
2. Cook for 5 minutes, until the onion is soft. Add the crushed tomatoes, diced tomatoes, basil, and oregano. Bring to a simmer.
3. Cook over medium heat until the sauce thickens slightly, stirring occasionally, about 14 minutes. Taste and adjust the seasoning with more salt and pepper as desired.

Recipe Notes

- *If purchasing pasta sauce, to keep the recipe Whole 30 compliant, ensure there are no added sugars or dairy in your sauce.
- Suggested brands I found online include Rao's Homemade Marinara Sauce, Mario Batali Tomato Basil Pasta Sauce, most Thrive Market sauces (aside from the vodka sauce, which has cream), and Trader Joe's Roasted Garlic Spaghetti Sauce (this is what I used).
- Be sure to double check the list of ingredients. You can also make the basic homemade spaghetti sauce I suggest above.

To freeze: Freeze with or without sauce for up to 2 months. Let thaw overnight in the refrigerator, and then reheat on the stove (with sauce to keep them from drying out).

Amount per serving (4 meatballs) — Calories: 185, Fat: 10g, Saturated Fat: 3g, Cholesterol: 23mg, Sodium: 236mg, Carbohydrates: 3g, Fiber: 1g, Protein: 26g

Mexican Chicken Soup

Thanksgiving | Christmas | New Year | Easter | Halloween

Prep Time: 5 minutes || Cook Time: 3 hours

Servings: 8

Calories: 125

Mexican Chicken Soup - Paleo, gluten-free and Whole friendly! An easy crock pot soup recipe that takes just 5 minutes of prep. This Mexican soup is packed with veggies and is healthy and delicious!

Ingredients

- 1 pound chicken breasts (boneless, skinless, about 2-3 large breasts)
- 32 ounces chicken broth (1 container)
- 29 ounces diced tomatoes (2 cans)
- 1 1/2 cups carrots (chopped)
- 1 1/2 cups celery (chopped)
- 1 cup onion (chopped)
- 1 cup red bell pepper (chopped)
- 1 cup cilantro (chopped)
- 1 1/2 cups water
- 1/4 cup tomato paste
- 2teaspoons minced garlic
- 1 teaspoon kosher salt
- 1 teaspoon cumin
- 1/2 teaspoon chili powder
- 1/2 lime (juiced)

Instructions

1. Combine all ingredients in a crock pot and cook on high for 3-4 hours or low for 6-8.
2. Cook until the chicken shreds easily and the vegetables are tender. Shred chicken and serve immediately.

Note: Sometimes I'll top with fresh cilantro, avocado and olives. This recipe makes a great freezer meal. Just place the leftovers in a Ziplock bag and place in the freezer. Thaw and warm before eating.

Calories: 125kcal | Carbohdrates: 12g | Protein: 14g | Fat: 2g | Cholesterol: 36mg | Sodium: 885mg | Potassium: 786mg | Fiber: 3g | Sugar: 6g | Vitamin A: 5110IU | Vitamin C: 49.3mg | Calcium: 74mg | Iron: 2.1mg

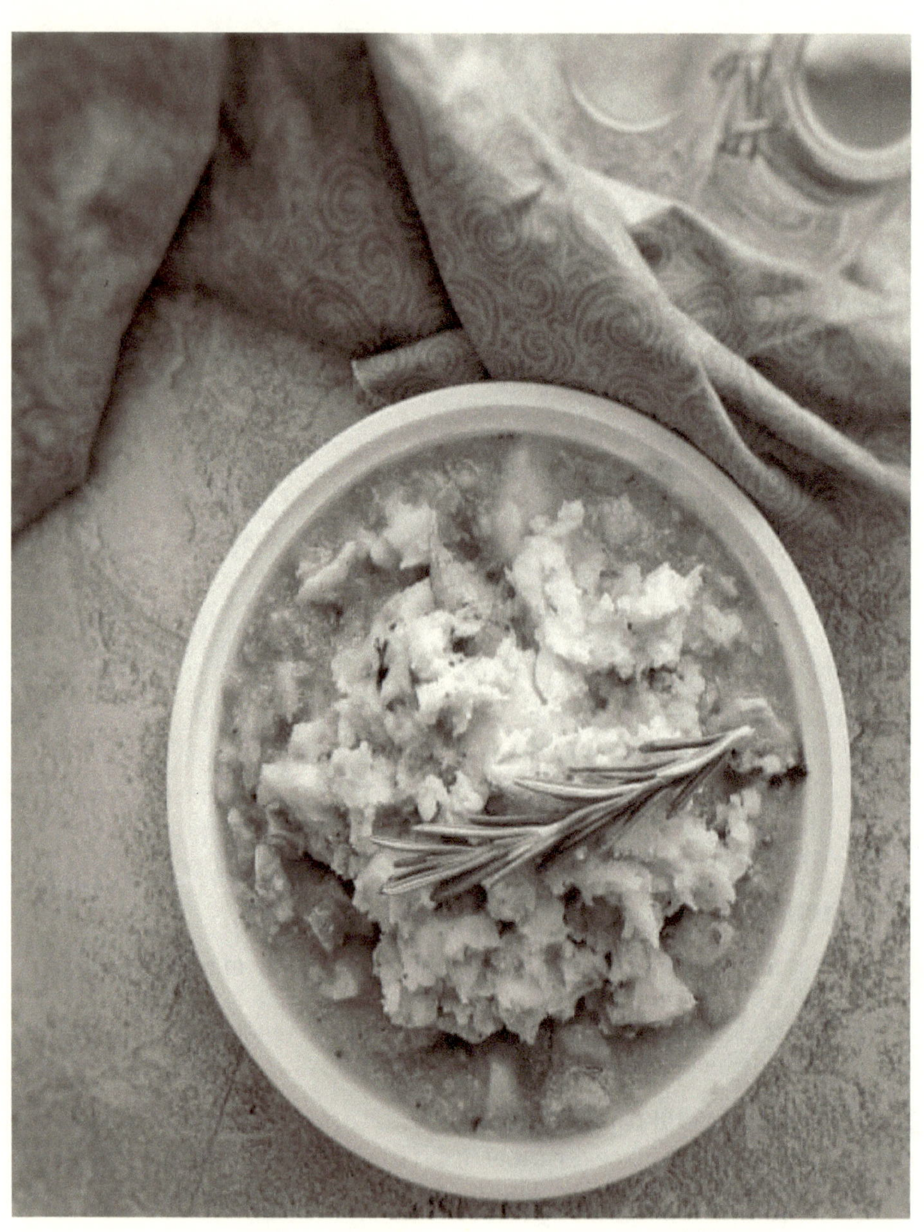

Chicken Pot Pie w/Mashed Potato Crust

Thanksgiving | Christmas | New Year | Easter | Halloween

Prep Time: 15 minutes || Cook Time: 1 hour

Yield: 4-6 servings

Serving Size: 2 cups

This chicken pot pie is hearty, warming, full of holiday flavor. Unlike traditional chicken pot pie, this recipe uses mashed potatoes as a crust to not only go on top, but also to thicken the dish without the use of flours or thickeners making it suitable for paleo and whole lifestyles.

Ingredients

For Pot Pie Filling

- 1 pound Chicken Breast Raw, diced small
- 1/2 cup Celery, diced
- 1/2 cup Carrots, diced (or frozen)
- 1 medium Onion, diced
- 2 tsp Garlic, minced
- 1 cup Green beans, cut and frozen
- 8oz can Coconut Milk
- 1-2 tbsp Poultry Seasoning
- 1 tsp Dried Rosemary
- 1 tbsp Ghee

For Mashed Potatoes

- 2 pounds Golden Potatoes
- 2 tbsp Ghee
- 1/2 tsp Garlic Powder
- Salt/Pepper to taste

Instructions

For Pot Pie Filling

1. In a medium sized pot, heat up 1 tbsp ghee over medium high heat.
2. Add carrots, celery, onion, garlic and saute for about 5 minutes or until vegetables soften.

3. Add in raw diced chicken breast along with green beans, poultry seasoning, rosemary, salt and pepper and saute in together for another 5 minutes or until all chicken is opaque.
4. Add in coconut milk, stir together and simmer over medium heat for about 20 minutes or until chicken is cooked all the way through.
5. The mixture of vegetables and chicken plus the liquid in the coconut milk should be enough to simmer without burning.
6. If the filling looks like there is not enough liquid to simmer, add water in 1/4 cup increments. It is also ok if the liquid has a thin broth consistency as potatoes will be added to thicken it.

For Mashed Potato Crust

1. In a large pot, boil 6-8 quarts of water.
2. Rinse then chop each potato into large chunks. I personally leave the skin on, but if you dont prefer it, peel each potato before boiling.
3. Boil potatoes for 25-35 minutes or until cooked through. The timing will depend on how big your potato pieces are.
4. Strain potatoes and add to a large bowl. Add salt, pepper, garlic powder and ghee.
5. Using a potato masher, mash potatoes into a rustic chunky mash being sure to make sure spices and ghee are evenly distributed.

To Bring It All Together

1. Take pot pie mixture off heat and stir in 1/3 of rustic potato mixture. This will thicken up the mixture without using any creams or thickeners. Feel free to use more or less potato to get the desired pot pie filling consistency.
2. Add filling to a large casserole dish or meal prep containers and top with the remaining mashed potato mix.
3. If you decide to put it in the casserole dish, you can place it under the broiler for a couple minutes to create a more of a brown crust effect on the top.

For Paleo Option: Use Avocado or Olive Oil in place of Ghee

Amount Per Serving: Calories: 290 Total Fat: 13g Saturated Fat: 9g Trans Fat: 0g Unsaturated Fat: 3g Cholesterol: 54mg Sodium: 128mg Carbohydrates: 29g Net Carbohydrates: 0g Fiber: 4g Sugar: 3g Sugar Alcohols: 0g Protein: 17g

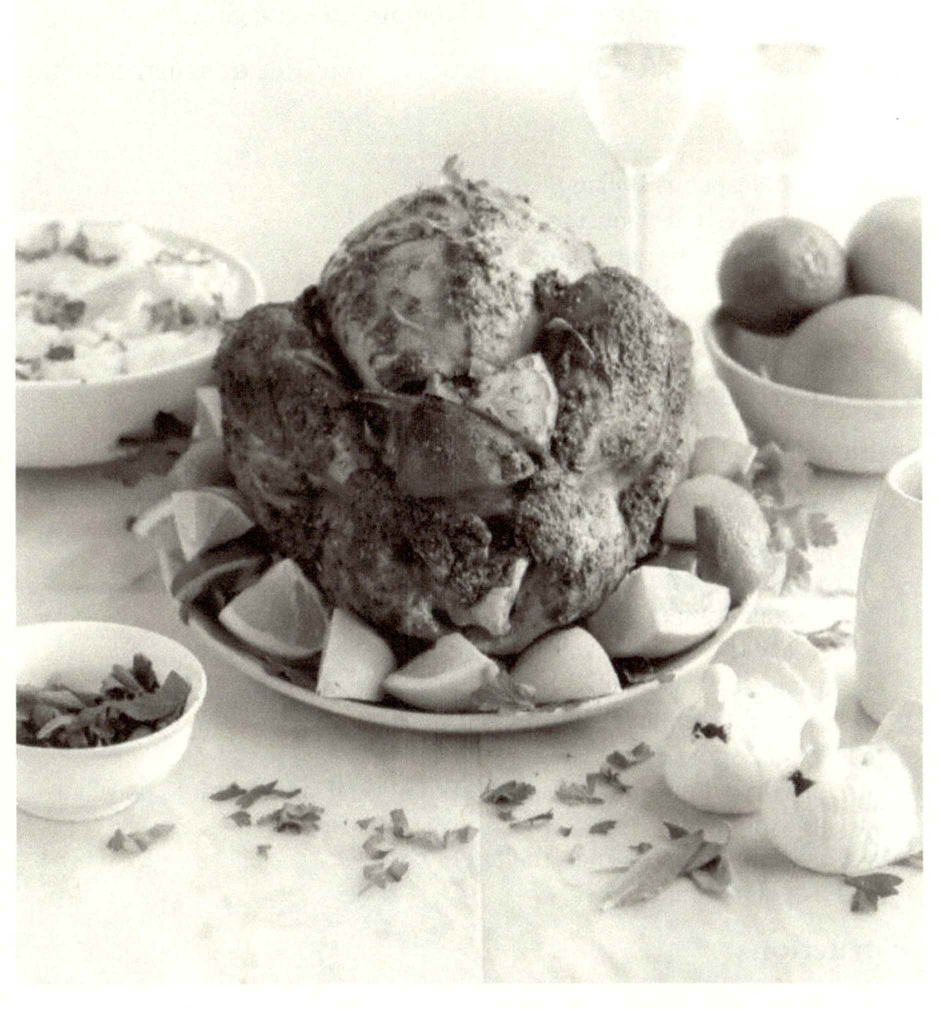

Herb-Citrus Roasted Thanksgiving Turkey

Prep Time: 30 minutes || Cook Time: 5 hour

Yield: 5 servings

Thanksgiving

The foolproof method for the most delicious Thanksgiving Day turkey!

Ingredients

- 18–22 pound turkey, rinse and remove neck and giblets)

Preheat oven to 375 (or the temp listed on your turkey's instructions)

Rub:

- 4 Tablespoons Italian Seasoning
- Tablespoon dry mustard
- 1 Tablespoons garlic powder
- 1 Ground black pepper
- 1 Tablespoon kosher salt
- olive oil
- 3–4 Tablespoons butter or ghee

Stuffing:

- 3 bay leaves
- 2 stalks of celery
- 1 onion, quartered
- 1 small orange, quartered
- 5 sage leaves
- 1 bunch of rosemary
- 1 bunch fresh thyme
- Baste Ingredients:
- 2/3 dry white wine (optional – don't use if you want it to be Whole 30 compliant)
- 2/3 cup butter or ghee, melted
- 2/3 cup orange juice

Instructions

1. Place turkey on rack in roaster or make rack with celery and carrots.
2. Rub 2 Tablespoons of seasoning inside.

3. Stuff cavity with Stuffing ingredients, above.
4. Rub enough olive oil over turkey and rub in.
5. Take the 3-4 Tablespoons of ghee or butter and rub all over turkey (or under skin, if desired).
6. Then take the remaining dry rub and rub all over turkey.
7. Loosely tent with foil.
8. Bake 3 1/2 – 4 hours, or until thermometer reads 180 degrees in thigh.
9. Baste every half hour with pan juice and Baste Ingredients.
10. Remove foil for last 30 minutes to brown turkey.

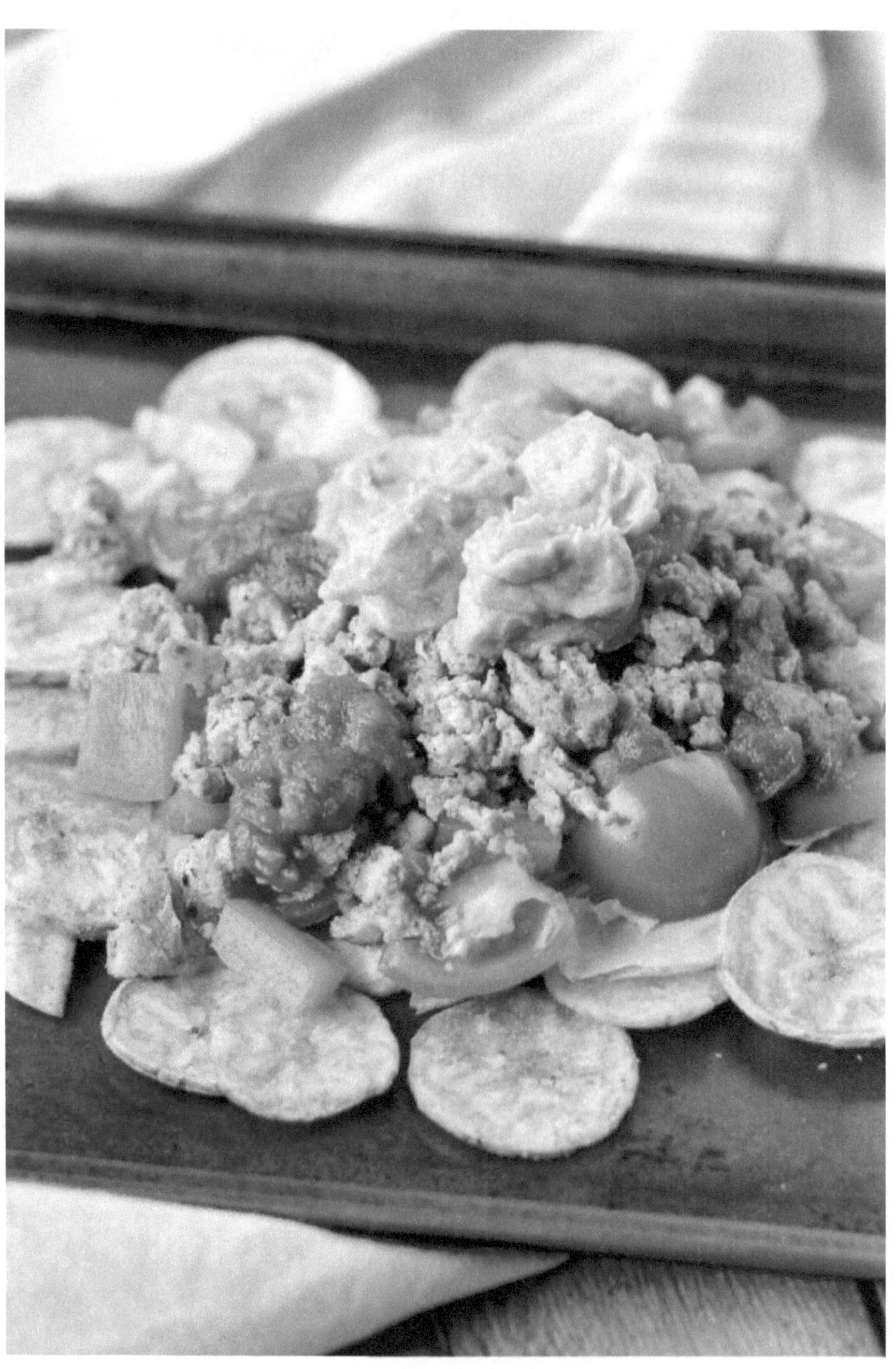

Ground Turkey Plantain Nachos

Ingredients

- 1 lb organic 93% lean ground turkey
- 2 TB of your favorite taco seasoning (this one is great and Whole 30-compliant)
- 1 6 oz bag of plantain chips (Inka are my favorites, or you can make your own!)
- 2 cups shredded lettuce

desired toppings: onions, peppers, tomatoes, salsa, guacamole, etc.

*The Whole 30 has since changed their program rules and chips are no longer allowed. Therefore, you will want to fry up your own plantain chips for these nachos!

Instructions

1. In a large skillet over medium heat, brown ground turkey until no longer pink. This will take approximately 10 to 15 minutes, depending on whether you have an electric or gas stove.
2. While the turkey is browning away, prepare your toppings. I shredded my lettuce, chopped onions and peppers, and sliced tomatoes.
3. Once the ground turkey is cooked through, add the taco seasoning and stir until well-combined.
4. Compile your nachos in the following order: plantain chips, shredded lettuce, onions, ground turkey, peppers, tomatoes, salsa, and guacamole (along with anything else that you love on top of nachos).

I like to eat these with a spoon because they do tend to get awfully messy!

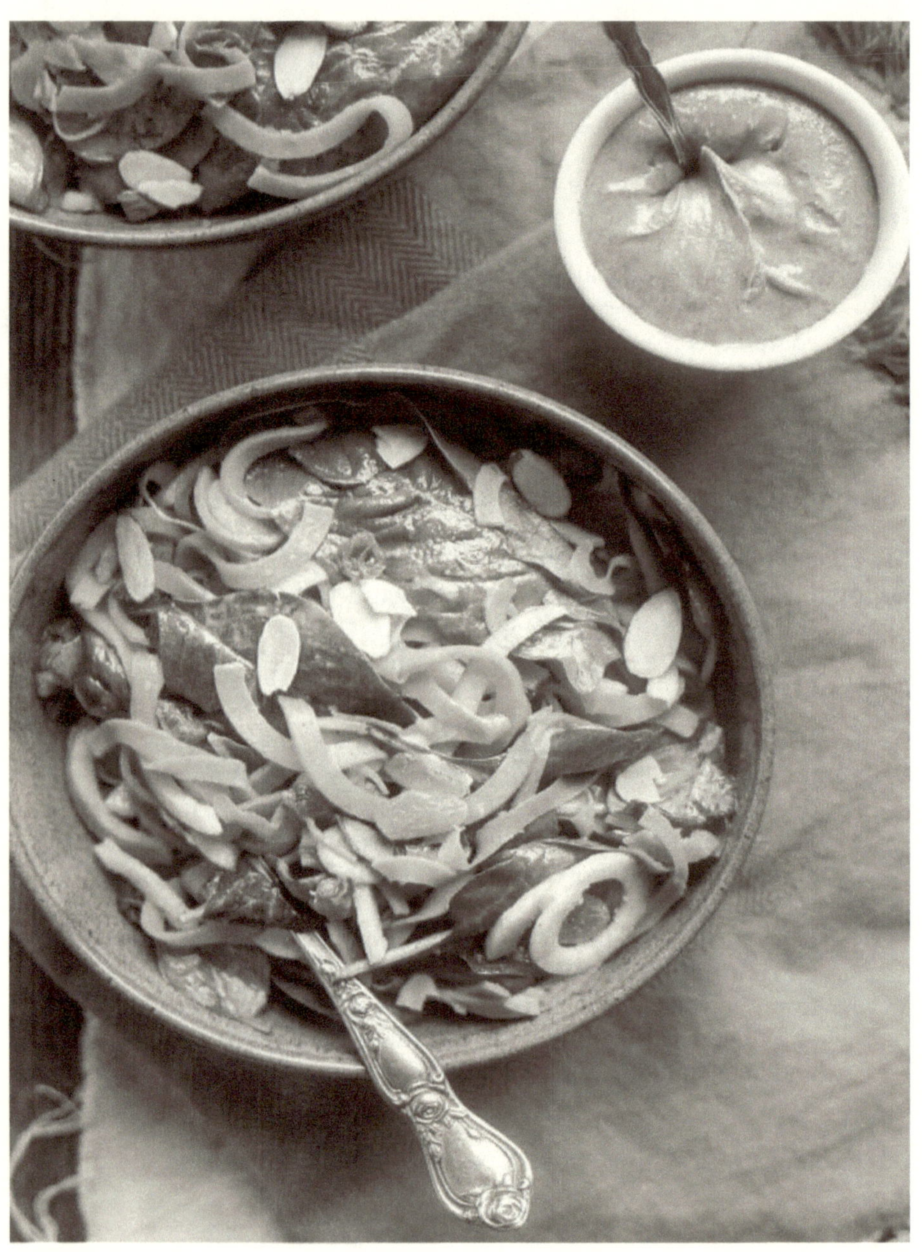

Sweet Potato Noodles and Apple Spinach Salad with Almond Dijon Vinaigrette

Prep Time 10 minutes || Cook Time 10 minutes

Course: Main Course, Salad

Servings 2

This vegan and whole spinach salad features sweet potato noodles, apples and a creamy almond Dijon vinaigrette for a healthy, weeknight meal!

Ingredients

For the salad:

- 3 Tbsp Sliced almonds
- 2 tsp Olive oil
- 1 Medium sweet potato spiralized with the 3mm blade, about 300g
- Sea Salt
- 1 Large Apple Spiralized with the 3mm blade I used fuji
- 3 Cups Spinach packed
- 3 Tbsp Golden raisins

For the vinaigrette:

- 2 Tbsp Pure apple juice
- 1 Tbsp Natural creamy almond butter
- 1 tsp Raw Apple cider vinegar
- 1 1/2 tsp Organic Dijon mustard make sure it doesn't have wine added
- 1/2 tsp Fresh ginger minced
- 1 Tbsp Olive oil
- Sea salt

Instructions

1. Preheat your oven to 350 degrees and place the almonds onto a small pan. Cook until lightly golden brown and toasted, about 7-10 mins. Watch them closely as they can burn quickly.
2. While the almonds cook, heat up the olive oil in a large pan on medium heat. Add the sweet potato noodles and cook, stirring frequently, until tender and wilted, about 7-10 mins. Season with sea salt.

3. Place the cooked sweet potato noodles into a bowl with the spiralized apple, spinach, golden raisins and add in the toasted almonds. Mix well.
4. Add the apple juice, almond butter and apple cider vinegar into a small, microwave-safe bowl and microwave for 30 seconds to soften to almond butter.
5. Add in the Dijon mustard and ginger. Whisk until smooth and well combined.
6. While whisking, add in the olive oil and whisk until smooth and creamy. Add a pinch of salt.
7. Pour the dressing over the salad and toss until evenly coated.
8. Divide between two plates and DEVOUR!

White Turkey Chili

Whole, Paleo

Prep Time: 10 mins//Cook Time: 30 mins

Thanksgiving | Christmas

Yield: 5

Category: Soup

Method: Pressure Cooker

A creamy, white soup with ground turkey, bacon and loads of flavor!

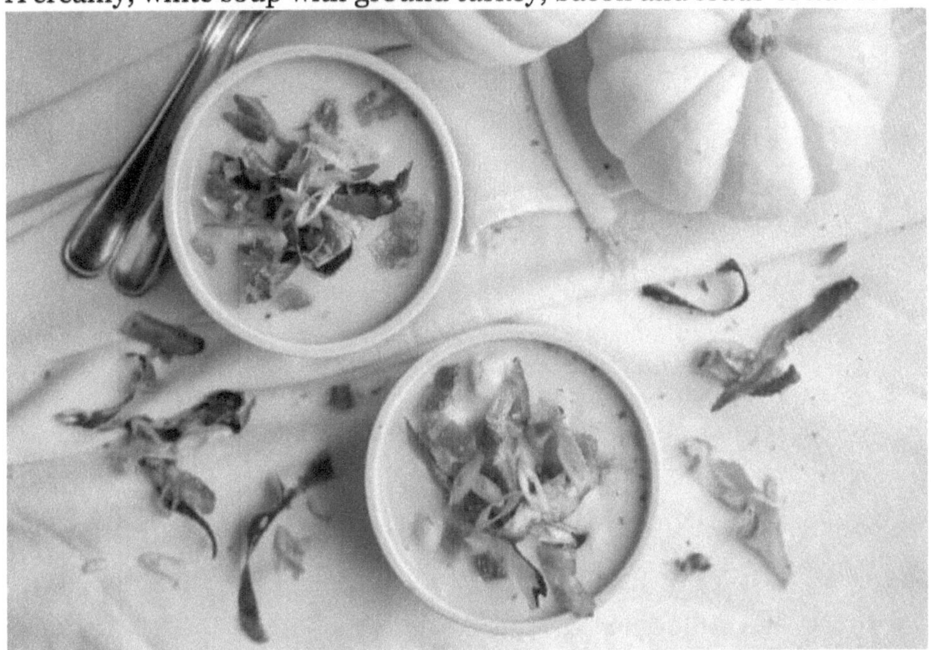

Ingredients

For Soup Base:

- 2 cups chopped leek whites
- 4–5 cups diced white sweet potatoes or 6 cups diced cauliflower
- 2 tbsp. bacon fat
- 1 tsp salt
- 1 tsp white pepper
- Pinch nutmeg
- 3 cups bone broth, more to taste
- 1 cup cashew or coconut cream

For Turkey

- 1–2lbs ground turkey
- ½ tsp salt
- ½ tsp mustard
- ½ tsp ground garlic
- ¼ cup minced leek greens
- 4 slices bacon

For Crispy Potato Skins *

- Sweet Potato Peels
- 1/4 cup coconut oil
- Skillet

Instructions

1. First begin by peeling your sweet potatoes and setting the skins aside, DO NOT DISCARD. Or dice your cauliflower.

START THE SOUP

2. Heat pressure cooker on saute mode.
3. Cut your bacon into 1/4 inch pieces.
4. Add it to the pot and cook until crispy.
5. In the meantime; slice your leeks until you hit the green part.
6. Once your bacon is crispy remove it from the pot and add in the leeks.
7. Saute until they begin to brown. Add in the sweet potato (or cauliflower)
8. Add in the broth, salt, white pepper and nutmeg.
9. Cancel saute function. Close the lid. Set to PRESSURE COOK: steam or vegetable mode.
10. During this time mix your ground turkey in a bowl with salt, mustard, ground garlic. Set aside.
11. Wash and mince the leek greens. Set aside.

MAKE CRISPY SKINS (IF USING POTATO)

1. Heat coconut oil in the skillet.
2. Line a plate with paper towel and set it close to the stove.
3. When a wooden spoon inserted in the oil sizzles, add in a handful of the potato skins.
4. Once they become golden brown (30-45 seconds) remove them with tongs and set on paper towel lined dish.
5. Repeat until all the skins are fried.

BACK TO THE SOUP

1. When the pressure cooker is done, release the pressure manually to speed up the process.
2. Then transfer all of the contents to a blender, carefully.
3. Place the insert back in the pot an heat on saute mode.
4. Add in the leek greens and ground turkey, saute until browned and cooked, about 5 minutes.
5. Stir often, you want to crumble the turkey with your spatula or spoon.
6. Blend the potato (or cauliflower) mix until smooth. Add in the cream. Blend again.
7. Pour your soup base into the pressure cooker and bring to a simmer with the turkey, this won't take but a minute or two.
8. If you want the soup thinner, add in more broth here. I like mine pretty thick!
9. Stir in MOST of the bacon, save some for garnish.
10. Serve soup. Top with crispy skins, bacon and green onion!
11. Boom! Delicious.
12. This will make a lot, about 5-6 bowls, which is about 8-10 cups.

Recipe Notes:

- AIP Modifications: Omit All The Seed Bases Spices Like Pepper, Nutmeg & Mustard.
- Use Horseradish, Ginger And A Little Cinnamon Instead.
- Use Coconut Cream Instead Of Cashew Cream.
- Ensure Your Bacon Is AIP Compliant.

Calories: 530, Fat: 34g, Carbohydrates: 17g, Fiber: 4g, Protein: 37g

Slow Cooker Turkey Breast

Paleo, Whole

Prep Time: 5 Minutes // Cook Time: 4 Hours 30 Minutes

Category: Main Course

Yield: 4

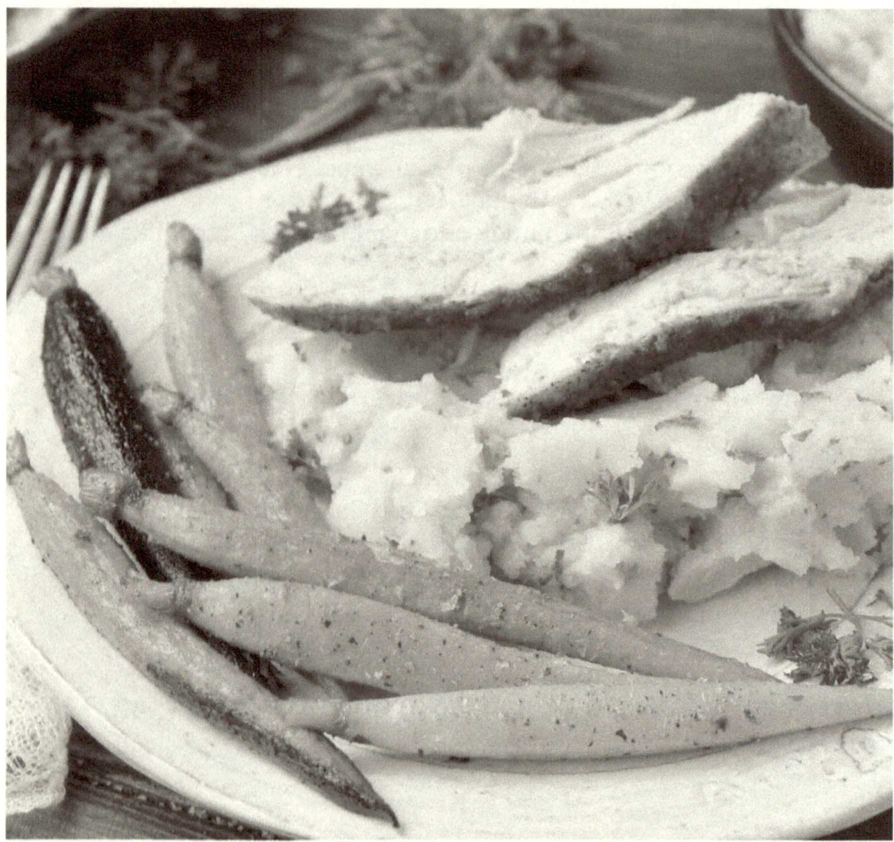

This Slow Cooker Turkey Breast is great for the holidays or as an easy dinner recipe year round! Add this to your small family holiday menu or make it as a nutritious meal. This is a Whole compliant and Paleo recipe.

Ingredients

- 1 teaspoon Garlic Powder
- 1 teaspoon Onion Powder
- 1/2 teaspoon Smoked Paprika
- 1/2 teaspoon Kosher Salt

- 1/2 teaspoon Ground Pepper
- Olive Oil
- 1 Sweet Onion, - cut into 1" rings
- 2 Lemons, - cut into 1/2" slices
- 3 Lb Halft Turkey Breast - skin on, bone in
- Fresh Rosemary
- Fresh Thyme
- Fresh Sage

Instructions

1. Mix together garlic powder, onion powder, paprika, salt and pepper. Set aside.
2. Drizzle olive oil inside a 6 quart slow cooker. Place the onions and lemons in a flat, even layer. Place the turkey breast on top, skin side up. Rub turkey breast with spices. Arrange fresh herbs around the turkey.
3. Cook on low for approximately 4½ hours. Begin checking internal temp every half hour at about the 3 hour mark. Once turkey reaches 165°F internal temp, remove from crockpot. Allow to sit for 10-15 minutes before slicing and serving.

Thai Chicken Soup Recipe

Prep Time 5 minutes // Cook Time 20 minutes

Servings 4 -5

Thanksgiving | Christmas | Halloween

Calories 190 kcal

Course: Main Course

Paleo, Whole, Dairy Free, Gluten Free

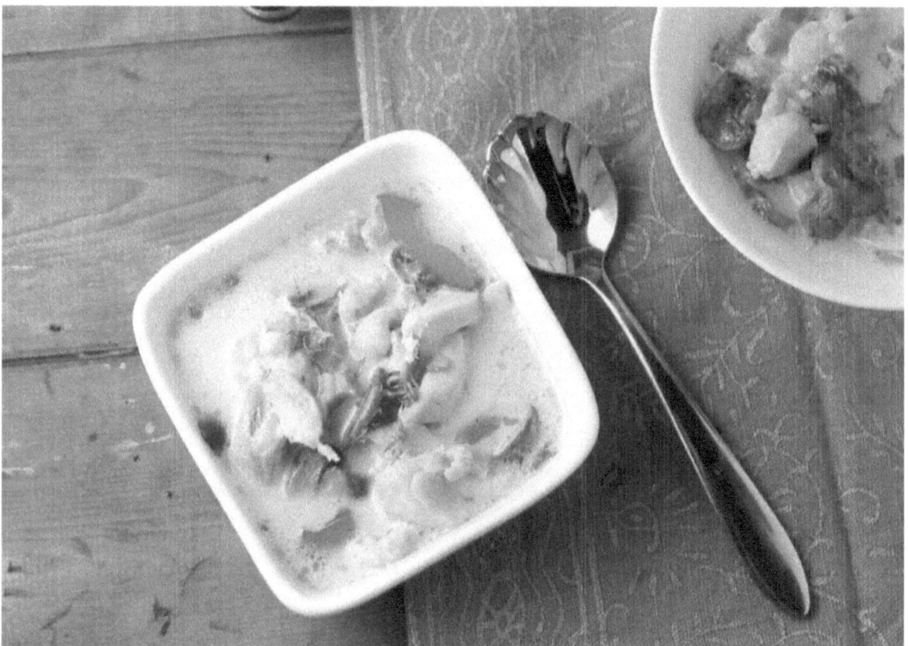

Ingredients

- 14 oz coconut milk this is my very favorite brand as it has no fillers/thickeners and amazing coconut cream!
- 2 cups chicken broth
- 6 slices FRESH ginger or galangal root about a quarter size each
- 1-2 lemongrass stalks cut into 3rds or 4ths, roughly smashed with a mallet or knife to release the flavor
- 1 pound boned and skinned chicken thighs cut into bite-size pieces
- cups sliced mushrooms I usually do a mix of cremini and shitake!
- 1 tablespoon Time juice or more taste
- 1 tablespoon fish sauce my favorite brand!!
- 1 teaspoon palm sugar or 4 drops liquid stevia, omit for Whole

- 1-3 teaspoons Thai Chile Garlic Sauce or paste or sriracha, check label for added sweetener
- 1/2 cup fresh cilantro finely minced
- 1 teaspoon sea salt to taste

Optional:

- Lots of veggies would make a good addition to this soup..I love sweet peppers!

Instructions

1. In a soup pot, bring the coconut milk, chicken broth, ginger, and lemongrass to a boil.
2. Add the chicken and mushrooms and simmer until cooked through, about 10 minutes.
3. Remove lemongrass and ginger slices.
4. Add the remaining ingredients, more or less as you prefer!! Enjoy!

Calories 190 Calories from Fat 54, Fat 6g9%, Saturated Fat 2g13%, Cholesterol 107mg36%, Sodium 1471mg64%, Potassium 569mg16%, Carbohydrates 7g2%, Sugar 4g4%, Protein 24g48%, Vitamin A 160IU3%, Vitamin C 10.9mg13%, Calcium 59mg6%, Iron 1.5mg8%

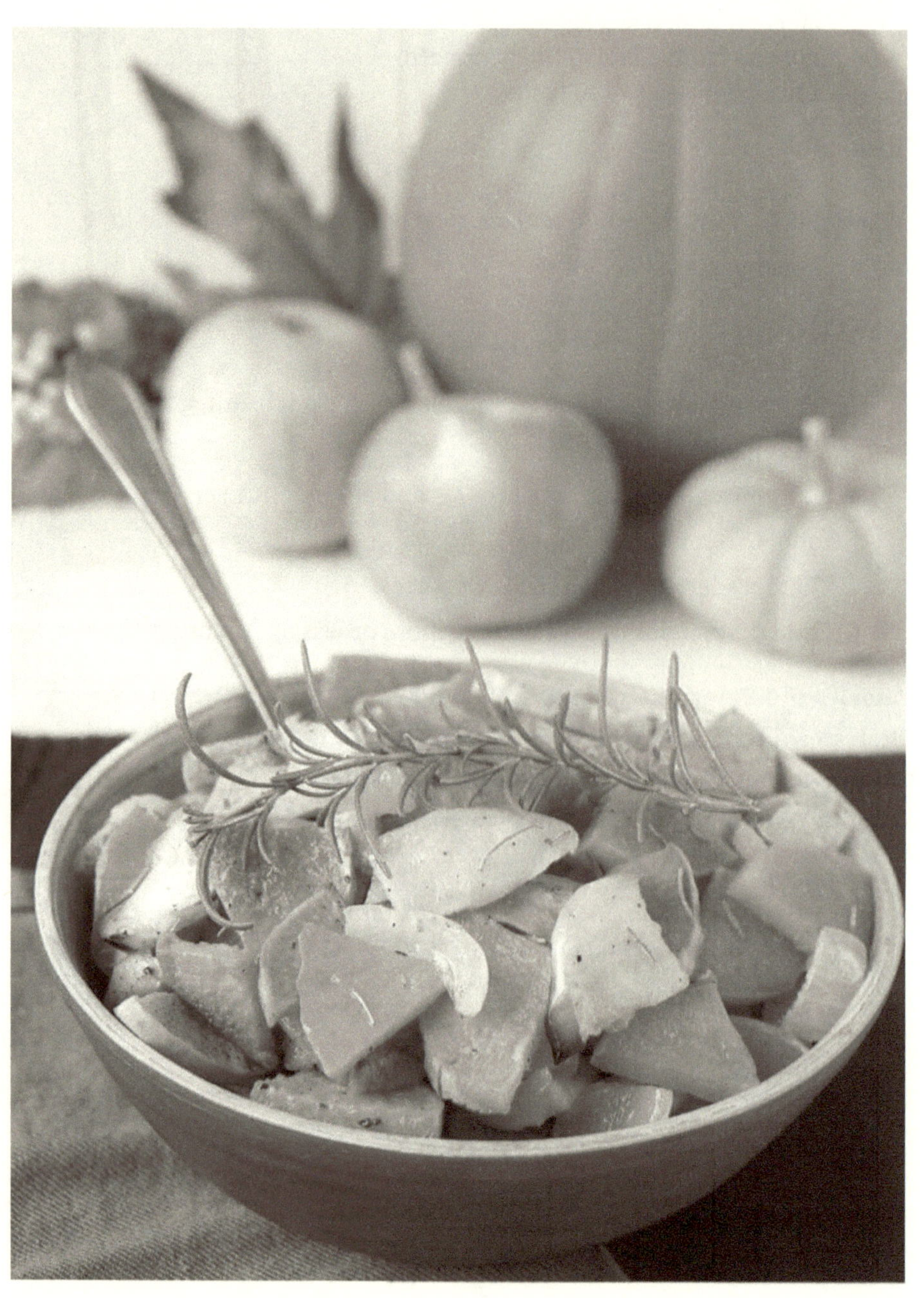

Roasted Sweet Potatoes, Squash, & Apples

Prep Time: 1 hr // Cook Time: 25 mins

Thanksgiving | Christmas | Halloween

Servings: 8 Servings

Course: Main dish

Ingredients

- 1 Extra Large Sweet Potato
- 1 Large Apple
- 1/2 Large Onion white or yellow
- 1 Honeynut Squash or 1/2 Butternut Squash
- Tbsp. Olive Oil
- 1 tsp. Dried Rosemary
- Salt and Pepper to taste

Instructions

1. Preheat oven to 400 degrees and line a baking sheet with parchment paper.
2. Chop sweet potatoes, squash, onion, and apple into bite-sized pieces and place on baking sheet.
3. Drizzle with olive oil and top with salt, pepper, and rosemary.
4. Bake for 20-25 minutes or until the vegetables are lightly browned on the edges.
5. Garnish with fresh rosemary

MAINTAIN AN ALLERGY FRIENDLY DURING HOLIDAY

The holidays are a time for celebrating and feasting. There's no reason you can't enjoy some great meals and stick to your Paleo diet. It's easy to lose sight of your health and nutrition goals this time of year. However, you don't want to start the new year having to begin from scratch. Let's look at some tips to maintain your healthy lifestyle and Paleo diet right through the holiday season.

HOST YOUR OWN PALEO-FRIENDLY DINNER

The simplest way to make sure a meal is Paleo is to cook it yourself. If you have a partner or friends who can help, so much the better. Another option is to make it a potluck where everyone brings a dish.

This isn't always practical for traditional family celebrations but it can be fun for parties among like-minded friends. In this case, even people who don't normally share the same diet can bring a dish that's appropriate for the occasion.

COMMUNICATE YOUR NEEDS

If you're attending a holiday dinner at someone else's home, let them know about your dietary restrictions. People are getting increasingly used to accommodating different diets such as vegan, gluten-free and, yes, Paleo.

Not all hosts are amenable to making special preparations for you. Your grandmother who's been making the turkey with stuffing the same way for 50 years might not want to alter her recipe just for you. In these cases, politely refuse anything that isn't suitable. If you know that the Paleo offerings will be limited, you can even bring something with you.

The key is to communicate in a non-confrontational manner with people so it doesn't look like you're insulting their cooking or trying to convert them to your diet.

STRATEGIC COMPROMISES

It's up to you whether to stay 100% compliant with your Paleo diet through the holidays or to make some exceptions. You might, for example, decide to compromise for one traditional family dinner and eat the non-Paleo stuffing, mashed potatoes, and dairy-rich desserts. Even then, you can always stick mainly to healthy foods and just take small samplings of everything else.

Most holiday dinners contain lots of dishes and people are unlikely to notice the quantity of each item you consume. Whether you decide to stay true to your Paleo diet or compromise for certain occasions, stick to your decision and don't feel guilty or apologize for it.

STAY ACTIVE

In addition to your diet, it's important to keep up with exercise during the holidays. If you're eating more than usual, you need to burn off those extra calories. Make sure you schedule workouts between all of your shopping, meals, and parties. If you don't currently have a regular workout schedule, the holidays are a good time to start. Many people join gyms in January to keep their New Year's resolutions but why not get a head start and join now?

ALLERGY-FRIENDLY HOLIDAY FOODS

Popular holiday dishes cover a wide spectrum when it comes to healthiness and Paleo-friendliness. In many cases, it all depends on how you prepare the food.

Here are some suggestions for food and snacks for the holidays.

1. **Grass-fed Meat and Poultry** -If you get your meats from organic sources, it's suitable for a Paleo diet. Typical supermarket meats, however, are usually from grain-fed animals and don't make the mark.
2. **Stuffing** – Many holiday meals are served with stuffing. Unfortunately, most stuffing is made with bread from grain flours. However, you can just as easily make stuffing with alternative ingredients such as mushrooms, almond flour, sweet potatoes, and other Paleo-friendly ingredients.
3. **Sweet Potatoes** – A delicious staple at all holiday meals. While white potatoes are not Paleo due to their starchiness and high-carb content, sweet potatoes are.
4. **Veggies** – Many vegetables are fine for a Paleo diet provided you don't cover them with butter or sauces containing dairy. Squash, broccoli, avocado, cabbage, mushrooms, and cauliflower are some nutritious vegetables to serve at your holiday meals. Dressings and sauces made from oil and vinegar are Paleo-friendly, as is salsa and any sauces made from almonds, walnuts, and other nuts.
5. **Dairy-free Pumpkin Pie** – Pumpkins are a healthy and tasty food that's often ruined with dairy and refined sugar. A pumpkin pie made with ingredients such as almond milk and sweet potatoes is just one example of a delicious Paleo dessert that's perfect for the holidays.

THE COMPLETE PALEO DIET FOOD LIST: WHAT TO EAT AND WHAT TO AVOID

Our comprehensive list of paleo diet foods tells you exactly what you can (and can't) eat on this prehistoric diet. Plan your shopping list with these paleo meats, vegetables, fruits, nuts, seeds, and oils, plus see a sample day of paleo eating.

The paleo diet is meant to mimic what our hunter-gatherer ancestors ate. But what foods should you eat to follow this diet and what foods do you want to avoid? If you're new to the paleo diet, knowing what to eat for breakfast, lunch and dinner can be hard. As with most diets, there are foods that are allowed and not allowed. Some foods also fall into a bit of a grey area and are sometimes allowed.

Our ultimate list of paleo-approved foods will help simplify your planning if you're dining out or cooking at home. Whether you're a beginner or just looking for a refresher on the rules, here's what you need to know to eat paleo.

What is the Paleo Diet?

The premise behind "eating paleo" is that the current Western diet is contributing to the rise of chronic diseases such as obesity, heart disease and cancer.

Paleo diet proponents claim, eating this way can reduce inflammation, improve workouts, increase energy, help with weight loss, stabilize blood sugar and even reduce the risk of chronic diseases.

The pros of paleo are that it focuses on increasing intake of whole foods, fruits and vegetables, lean proteins and healthy fats and decreasing consumption of processed foods, sugar and salt. For those looking to eat a more well-rounded diet, these "guidelines" sound familiar and altogether healthy.

However, the paleo diet also advocates cutting out grains, dairy and legumes, and this has caused controversy among scientists. These foods, despite what paleo advocates claim, are healthful and can be good sources of fiber, vitamins and minerals.

Foods You Can Eat on the Paleo Diet

In short, if your ancestors could hunt or gather it, it is allowed on the paleo diet. This includes:

- Grass-fed meat: choosing grass-fed is healthier for you, the environment and closer to what our ancestors ate.
- Fish and seafood: choose wild-caught
- Fresh fruits and veggies
- Eggs
- Nuts and seeds
- Healthy oils (olive, walnut, flaxseed, macadamia, avocado, coconut)
- Meat & Seafood

Most meat and seafood fits on a paleo diet. Meat is a source of lean protein, and protein is the building block of all cells and tissues.

Protein also helps keep you full. Watch out for pre-marinated meats that may contain added sugar. Common meat and seafood choices include:

Paleo Meat & Seafood

- Chicken
- Beef
- Salmon
- Tuna
- Pork
- Bacon
- Cod
- Turkey

Grass-fed meat is recommended on the paleo diet because it is leaner than meat from grain-fed animals and has more omega-3 fatty acids, the healthy fats that reduce inflammation in the body and protect your heart.

A typical American diet is high in saturated and trans fats and lower in healthy poly- and monounsaturated fats, hence the paleo diet's emphasis on grass-fed meats.

Look for chicken raised without antibiotics and try to source your meat from a local farm to learn more about how it was raised.

Choosing wild seafood over farm-caught may help boost your omega-3 intake too. That's not always the case, but look for wild salmon and other sustainably-caught seafood when you're eating paleo.

Fruits & Vegetables

The Paleo Diet: Is Eating Like Our (Very Distant) Ancestors Really a Good Idea?

There is little argument over the health benefits of fruits and vegetables. They are chock-full of vitamins, minerals, fiber and antioxidants. The only caveat for paleo dieters is that some vegetables are starchy (e.g., potatoes) and some fruits are higher in sugar (e.g., bananas).

So, if you are trying to lose weight or watch your blood sugar levels, eat these in moderation. In fact, potatoes are banned from some strict versions of the diet.

Many paleo followers wonder if bananas are paleo, because of their higher sugar content. They are considered paleo. One medium banana has 100 calories, 3 grams of fiber and 25 grams of carbohydrate. Bananas are a good source of potassium and they are an unprocessed, whole food.

The key to remember with eating paleo is that you want your diet to contain unprocessed, whole foods so fruits and vegetables should make up a bulk of your diet. Frozen vegetables without added sauce, are also allowed on a paleo diet.

Examples of produce to eat on a paleo diet:

- Cauliflower
- Broccoli
- Brussels sprouts
- Sweet potatoes
- Butternut squash
- Cabbage
- Spinach
- Paleo Fruits
- Apples

- Berries: including blackberries, blueberries and strawberries
- Melon
- Grapes
- Bananas
- Citrus fruits
- Peaches
- Plums
- Eggs

Eggs are allowed because they are high in protein, B vitamins, minerals and antioxidants. They are also affordable and easy to prepare. Buy "organic" and "cage-free" eggs for a higher omega-3 content than eggs from chickens raised in cages.

Nuts & Seeds

Nuts and seeds are full of healthy fats, fiber and protein. Plus, they were foraged in prehistoric times, so you can load up your cart with them. Keep in mind that peanuts are not considered paleo because they are technically legumes.

Paleo Nuts & Seeds

- Almonds
- Cashews
- Pistachios
- Walnuts
- Macadamia nuts
- Pecans
- Hazelnuts
- Pine nuts
- Brazil nuts
- Pumpkin seeds (pepitas)
- Chia seeds
- Sunflower seeds
- Flax seeds
- Healthy Oils
- roasted cauliflower and walnut dip

Oils

The Paleo Diet Movement, breaks down which oils are healthy on the paleo diet: olive, walnut, flaxseed, macadamia, avocado and coconut oils are all allowed because they were gathered directly from the plant.

While our hunter-gatherer ancestors probably did not consume flaxseed oil, it is allowed because of its content of high alpha-linolenic acid (ALA), a type of heart-healthy, anti-inflammatory omega-3 fatty acid.

Paleo Oils

- Olive oil
- Walnut oil
- Flaxseed oil
- Macadamia oil
- Avocado oil
- Coconut oil

Foods You Should Avoid on the Paleo Diet

If you are following a strict paleo diet, you should avoid the following foods. These foods are not permitted on the paleo diet:

- Cereal grains
- Legumes (peanuts, beans, lentils, tofu)
- Refined sugar
- Processed foods
- Soda & sweetened beverages
- Refined vegetable oils
- Salt
- Artificial sweeteners
- Grains

Say goodbye to cereal, crackers, rice, pasta, bread and beer. Yes, beer. All grains are forbidden on the paleo diet.

Why? First, grains are a product of modern agriculture; cavemen didn't nosh on bread. Second, grains are high in carbohydrates, which can spike your blood sugar.

Paleo critics point out that not all grains are created equal-whole grains do not spike your blood sugar as much as refined grains. Even so, paleo dieters still steer clear of grains because they contain different compounds and proteins like gluten, lectins and phytates, which they claim cause inflammation in the body and block other nutrients from being absorbed. Paleo critics say these compounds are not a problem unless you have an allergy or sensitivity.

Legumes

Legumes are members of a large family of plants that have a seed or pod. This category includes all beans, peas, lentils, tofu and other soy foods, and peanuts. This also includes peanut butter and soy sauce. Legumes are not allowed on paleo because of their high content of lectins and phytic acid. Similar to grains, this is a point of controversy in the scientific community. In fact, lots of research supports eating legumes as part of a healthy diet because they are low in fat and high in fiber, protein and iron.

Processed Foods

Processed foods are full of the rest of the no-no's on the paleo diet: refined sugars, salt, refined vegetable oils and artificial sweeteners. Our ancestors didn't eat these foods. Plus, there is little argument in the scientific community that refined sugars and excess salt contribute to obesity, high blood pressure and heart disease.

There is some disagreement, however, over vegetable oils and artificial sweeteners. The American Heart Association recommends consuming corn, safflower and canola oils, but paleo plans say these are "not allowed" because of the ratio of omega-6 to omega-3 fatty acids and the way the oils are processed.

The U.S. Food and Drug Administration (FDA) condones artificial sweeteners as safe to consume, but they are not allowed on paleo since they are a man-made, processed food. Plus, although artificial sweeteners lower calories in food, research shows they can still cause us to crave sweets and that they can be harmful to our gut bacteria.

Foods You Can Sometimes Eat on the Paleo Diet

Dairy

A strict paleo diet does not allow dairy products because hunter-gatherers did not milk cows. This includes milk, butter, yogurt, sour cream, and cheese.

However, some paleo dieters say dairy is OK, especially if it is grass-fed because grass-fed butter, for example, has more omega-3s. Fermented dairy products like kefir are also OK for some paleo eaters because they have a lower content of lactose and casein, the two concerns paleo dieters have with dairy.

If you prefer to avoid dairy on the paleo diet, you can substitute non-dairy products made with coconut milk, almond milk, and cashew milk.

Starchy Vegetables & High-Sugar Fruits

This is a gray area. Sugary fruits and starchy vegetables (potatoes, squash, beets) can spike your blood sugar more than berries and spinach. That's why these are OK in moderation and are best to minimize if you are trying to lose weight, according to paleo experts.

Alcohol

Alcohol is a no-no if you are strict paleo. Beer is made from grains, and liquor also contains traces of gluten. But, good news for cider-lovers: most hard ciders are gluten-free, so they are allowed.

Check the label to be sure. Red wine is more accepted in the paleo community because it contains the antioxidant resveratrol, but sorry chardonnay lovers, white wine is technically not allowed.

CHEESE AND CONDINMENT

The Mozzarella Cheese Recipe

Prep Time: 2 mins // Cook Time: 8 mins

Thanksgiving | Christmas | New Year

Course: Appetizer

Servings: 8

Calories: 98 kcal

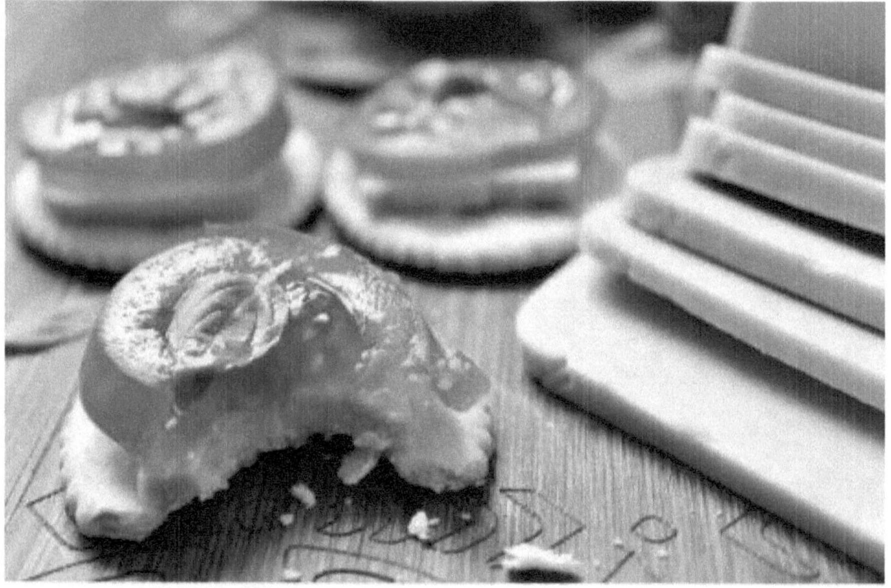

A delicious vegan mozzarella recipe that melts made with coconut milk

Ingredients

- 1 can coconut milk full fat
- 1/2 cup hot water
- 1 tsp salt
- 1 tbsp. nutritional yeast
- 2 tbsp. agar powder
- 1 tsp tapioca flour
- 1/4 tsp garlic powder minced

Instructions

1. Prepare cheese molds by spraying a glass bowl or container with spray oil or rub any neutral flavored oil on the molds to prevent sticking. (Recipe will make about 2 cups of cheese).

2. Pour the can of coconut milk into a saucepan.
3. Put 1/2 cup of hot water into the empty coconut milk can to melt all the remaining coconut milk and add the water to the pan.
4. Add all remaining ingredients to the saucepan and stir with a whisk.
5. Turn heat on to medium and stir frequently until it boils.
6. Turn down the heat until the cheese sauce is just barely boiling and stir constantly for 6 minutes until it is very smooth.
7. Immediately pour into the prepared cheese molds.
8. Let it cool with the lid off for about 15 minutes at room temperature, then transfer to the refrigerator for at least 2 hours to firmly set.
9. Once the cheese is cooled completely, cover and store in the refrigerator in a sealed for up to a week.

Recipe Notes

1. To make this cheese able to melt and better for use on pizza or grilled cheese, add 2 additional tablespoons of tapioca starch.
2. For best results when melting, let the cheese heat up to room temperature before cooking.
3. This cheese melts beautifully in the microwave too!
4. For a firmer cheese, leave out the tapioca starch from the recipe.

Calories 98Calories from Fat 90

Fat 10g15%, Saturated Fat 9g56%, Sodium 297mg13%, Potassium 123mg4%, Carbohydrates 2g1%, Protein 1g2%, Vitamin C 0.5mg1%, Calcium 9mg1%, Iron 1.6mg9%

The Cheddar Cheese Recipes

Prep Time: 5 minutes // Cook Time: 6 minutes

Thanksgiving | Christmas | New Year

Servings: 8

Calories: 81kcal

Course: Snack

Thanksgiving/Christmas/New Year

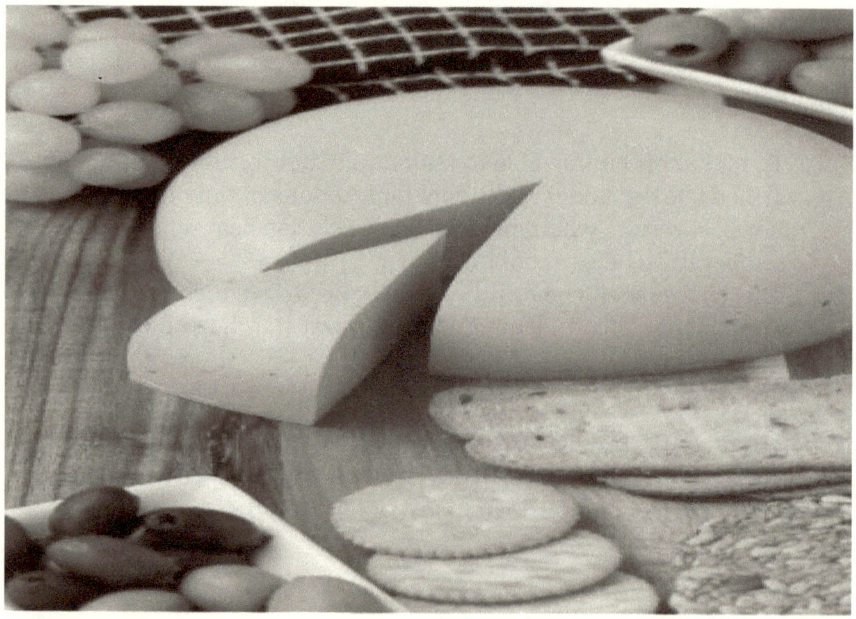

An easy way to make homemade vegan cheddar without nuts, gluten, or dairy.

Ingredients

- 2 cups soy milk or any other PLAIN plant-based milk
- 1/4 cup nutritional yeast
- 3 tbsp. refined coconut oil or any neutral flavored oil
- 2 tbsp. agar powder (or 6 tbsp. agar flakes)
- 1 tsp salt
- 1 tsp lemon juice
- 1/8 tsp turmeric

Add for cheddar that melts and stretches "optional*

- 2 tbsp. + 1 tsp. tapioca starch (aka tapioca flour) (optional)

Add after cooking:

- 2 tbsp. warm water

- 1 tbsp. white miso paste (or any mild flavored miso)
- 1 squirt spray oil (to coat the cheese mold)

Instructions

1. Prepare a cheese mold by spraying a smooth glass container with a little oil.
2. Pour all of the ingredients except for the water and miso into a medium sized saucepan.
3. Stir the ingredients and turn on the heat to medium.
4. Cook your cheese sauce until it has slowly boiled for 6 minutes while stirring frequently. (It needs to boil for 6 minutes to fully melt and activate the agar agar).
5. Mix the miso and water until the miso is dissolved completely and pour it into the cheese sauce.
6. Stir the cheese sauce until the miso in incorporated.
7. Pour the cheese into the chosen mold.
8. Cool for about 15 minutes on the countertop and then put it in the refrigerator uncovered for 2 more hours until it cools and sets completely.
9. Serve or put in a sealed container in the fridge for later.

Recipe Notes

1. Once the cheese sauce begins to boil, turn the heat down so that it is bubbling, but not so hot that it will burn.
2. Be sure to stir the cheese sauce very frequently so it doesn't' burn.
3. Simmer the cheddar cheese for 6 minutes to melt the agar and allow it to bind completely with the ingredients.
4. Adding the miso at the end makes it so you do not kill the beneficial probiotic in the miso.
5. Leave out the tapioca starch if you want a firm sliced cheese for crackers or just eating cold.

For Cheddar that melts:

1. Use the tapioca starch if you are using this cheese make anything hot like a grilled cheese where you would want it to melt.
2. I have found that exactly 2 tablespoons plus an additional 1 teaspoon of tapioca starch is the perfect amount to make it melt the best.

Note: your cheese will be softer with the tapioca starch added.

Amount Per Serving (0.25 cup); Calories 81Calories from Fat 54

Fat 6g9%, Saturated Fat 4g25%, Sodium 400mg17%, Potassium 117mg3%, Carbohydrates 3g1%, Sugar 1g1%, Protein 2g4%, Vitamin A 240IU5%, Vitamin C 4.6mg6%, Calcium 85mg9%, Iron 0.4mg2%

The Vegan Parmesan Cheese

Prep Time: 5 mins

Thanksgiving | Christmas | New Year | Easter

Yield: ~1 and 1/4 cup

Serving Size: 1 Tbsp.

Category: Savory, Side

Simple 4-ingredient vegan Parmesan cheese! Ideal to sprinkle over absolutely everything, but especially on pastas and vegan pizzas.

Ingredients

- 1 cup (150g) Raw Cashews
- 1/4 cup (15g) Nutritional Yeast
- 1/2 tsp Garlic Powder
- 3/4 tsp Sea Salt

Instructions

1. Add the ingredients to the food processor and pulse it on the S blade until it reaches a fine consistency.
2. Keep it in a sealable jar in the refrigerator where it will keep for weeks!
3. Sprinkle it on pastas, pizzas, casseroles, salads and anywhere else you can possibly think of!

Calories: 48Sugar: 0.5gSodium: 111mgFat: 3.5gSaturated Fat: 0.6gCarbohydrates: 2.8gFiber: 0.5gProtein: 2g

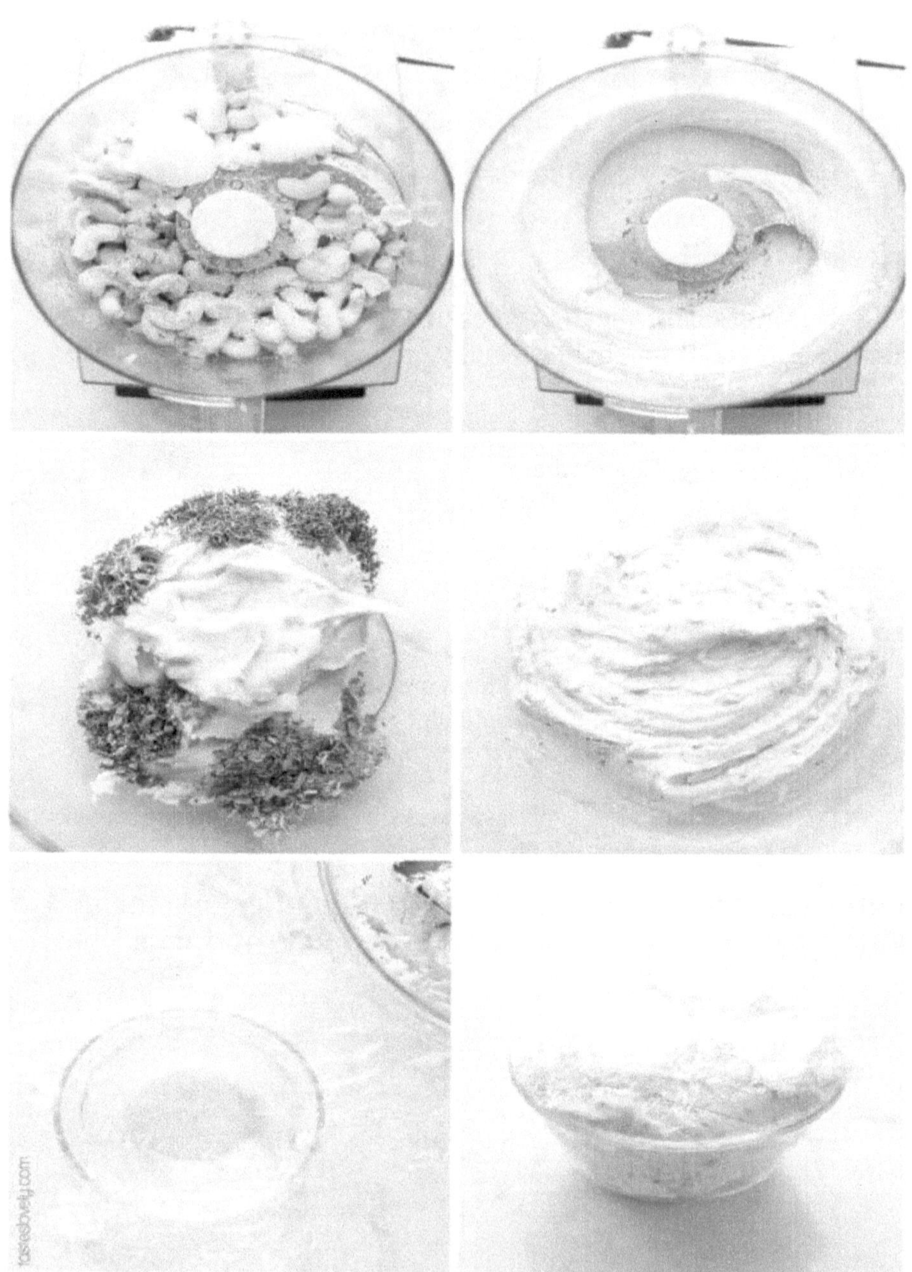

Herbed cashew cheese (paleo + keto)

Prep Time: 5 minutes // Cook Time: 10 minutes

Thanksgiving | Christmas | New Year | Easter

Yield: 7

This low-carb, paleo, and vegan nacho cheese sauce is rich, creamy, cheesy, and comforting. Even if you CAN have dairy, this is sure to be a hit and having you wanting more.

5 from 2 votes

Ingredients

- 1 cup raw cashews, soaked in water overnight and drained
- 2 tablespoons refined coconut oil
- 1 clove of garlic, grated
- 1/2 teaspoon lemon zest (about half a lemon)
- 2 tablespoons lemon juice (about half a juicy lemon)
- 1/2 teaspoon kosher salt
- 1/4 teaspoon white pepper (or black pepper works too)
- 1 teaspoon dried basil leaves
- 1 teaspoon dried chives
- 1/2 teaspoon dried parsley
- 1/4 teaspoon dried dill
- 1/4 teaspoon dried thyme
- Almond pulp crackers or raw vegetables for serving

Instructions

1. In your food processor with the S-blade attachment, add the soaked cashews, coconut oil, garlic, lemon zest, lemon juice, salt and pepper.
2. Blend until completely smooth, at least 10 minutes. Scrape down the sides of the bowl 2 or 3 times.
3. Transfer the cashew cheese to a mixing bowl. Add the dried herbs and mix completely.
4. Line a 6-ounce custard cup (or any small bowl) with saran wrap. Scoop the herbed cashew cheese into the custard cup, and fold the saran over the top. Place in the fridge for at least 2 hours to set.
5. Serve cold with almond pulp crackers or raw vegetables.
6. Will keep refrigerated for 7 days

Raspberry Jelly (sugar free jam)

Prep Time 5 minutes//Cook Time 20 minutes

Thanksgiving | Christmas | New Year | Easter

Makes: 1 cup or 16 servings (1 tbsp each)

Each tbsp is 1 net carb.

Calories 5kcal

Servings 16

A delicious low carb sugar-free raspberry jelly and the perfect low-sugar spread for low carb breads, low carb muffins and more!

Ingredients

- 6 ounces raspberries
- 1/2 cup water
- 1/4 cup Sukrin :1 (or Swerve or honey for Paleo)
- 1 tbsp lemon juice
- 3/4 tsp gelatin (Knox) (you may need more grass fed gelatin)
- stevia glycerite to taste

Instructions

1. Put the lemon juice in a small measuring cup or ramekin and sprinkle the gelatin over.
2. Add the raspberries, water, and Sukrin :1 to a small pot over medium heat. Bring to a low boil and turn heat down to medium low.
3. Simmer the raspberries for 20 minutes, stirring every few minutes. They will totally break apart.
4. Break up the gelatin and add to the raspberries, stirring to dissolve. Taste and adjust sweetness with the stevia glycerite. Cool.
5. Transfer the raspberry jelly/jam to a clean container and refrigerate overnight to gel. Keeps up to 1 week.

Notes

-Use 1 tsp of gelatin if using Great Lakes Grass Fed Beef Gelatin.

Serving: 1tbsp | Calories: 5kcal | Carbohydrates: 1g | Fiber: 1g

Homemade Almond Milk

Thanksgiving | Christmas | New Year | Easter

Servings: 4 cups

Ingredients

- 1 cup of almonds
- 4 cups of filtered water

Instruction

1. Soak the almonds in the water overnight
2. Drain and rinse the almonds
3. Add almonds and water into the high-speed blender and process for 30 sec-1 minute
4. Strain the milk through a nut bag, strainer, or cottage cheese fabric, or any other fabric
5. Store the milk in the fridge for up to 48 hours for a nice flavor!
6. Enjoy!

Italian Dressing Recipe

Thanksgiving | Christmas | New Year | Easter

Prep Time: 4 Mins || Cook Time: 5 Mins

Yield: 16 spoons

Recipe Type: side

An easy zesty Italian vinaigrette—just throw a few ingredients in a jar and shake.

Ingredients

- 1 tablespoon chopped fresh herbs - I used Italian flat leaf parsley
- 1 teaspoon dried oregano
- 1 clove garlic minced with a garlic press
- 1/2 teaspoon sea salt or more to taste
- 1/4 teaspoon fresh cracked black pepper
- 1/4 cup red wine vinegar
- 3/4 cup organic extra virgin olive oil

Instructions

1. Shaking Method: Add all ingredients to a jar or bottle with a tight-fitting lid and shake vigorously until well combined.
2. Whisking Method: Add all ingredients to a mixing bowl and whisk until the ingredients come together.
3. Taste and adjust seasonings if needed.

Calories: 91kcal | Fat: 10g | Saturated Fat: 1g | Sodium: 73mg | Potassium: 2mg | Vitamin A: 50IU | Vitamin C: 0.2mg | Calcium: 4mg | Iron: 0.1mg

Nut Cream Cheese

Thanksgiving | Christmas | New Year | Easter

Prep Time: 2 days

Servings: 3

Okay! So I made Coconut cream Cheese , I made Ricotta Cheese and Now this is my NUT Cream Cheese, which is really delicious and doesn't taste like Nuts at all! This can be made with ANY type of Nuts you like! So today I've decided to make my cream cheese with Cashews!

Ingredients:

- 1 1/2 Cups Soaked Raw Cashews
- 1 1/2 Tbl Apple Cider Vinegar
- 1 1/2 Tbl Fresh Lemon Juice
- 3 Tbl Spring Water
- (After this is done, you can add your own Herbs, Sweetener, and Vanilla etc.) Depending on what you're going to use the cream cheese for).

Instructions:

1. You must soak the cashews for about 24 hours.
2. After it's been soaked, Drain, Strain and rinse.
3. Blend all the Ingredients in blender till nice and smooth.
4. (If you want a Creamy cheese then double up on your cheese cloth)
5. Pour everything in your cheese cloth.
6. Hang and leave in a warm dark place for at least 24 hours.
7. Remove and Enjoy!

Ricotta Cheese

Prep Time: 15 Mins // Cook Time: 35 Mins

Thanksgiving | Christmas | New Year | Easter

Servings: 6

This REALLY tastes just like RICOTTA CHEESE!!! First off make sure you buy the Coconut creamer for this recipe which will do wonders in this recipe or if you can't find… you can use coconut Milk which will work but will make it a little watery so best to get the creamer.

Ingredients:

- 4 Cups Coconut Creamer
- 1 Tsp. Lemon Juice
- 2 Tsp. Olive Oil
- 1 Tsp. Pink Himalayan Salt
- 4 Tbl Agar Flakes or 2 Tsp. Agar Powder
- 1 1/2 Tsp. Garlic powder
- 1 Tsp. Onion Powder

Instructions:

1. In a sauce pan, mix all the ingredients together.
2. Stirring consistently bring the mixture to a boil.
3. Put temperature to low, let it simmer for about 7 minutes.
4. Remove from heat and let it cool for 10-12 minutes.
5. Transfer to a sealed glass container and refrigerate for a few hours to set.
6. Then you are going to place it in a food processor and pulse until you get the desired consistency

Enjoy!

2 Ingredient Dairy Free Sweetened Condensed Milk

Ingredients

- 1 Can Full-Fat Coconut Milk 13.5 oz
- 1/3 Cup Gentle Sweet or the equivalent of your favorite powdered sweetener

Instructions

1. In a large skillet/frying pan, combine coconut milk and Gentle Sweet.
2. Bring to a boil, and turn down heat to a simmer.
3. Simmer, stirring occasionally, for 20-25 minutes, or until the liquid has reduced by about half.

Notes

My milk only took about 20-25 minutes to condense, but yours may or may not take longer. I have found (by experience) that the larger the surface of the pan (think frying pan), the faster the milk will condense. It should be slightly thick and gooey when it is finished. It will also continue to thicken as it cools.

BREAKFAST

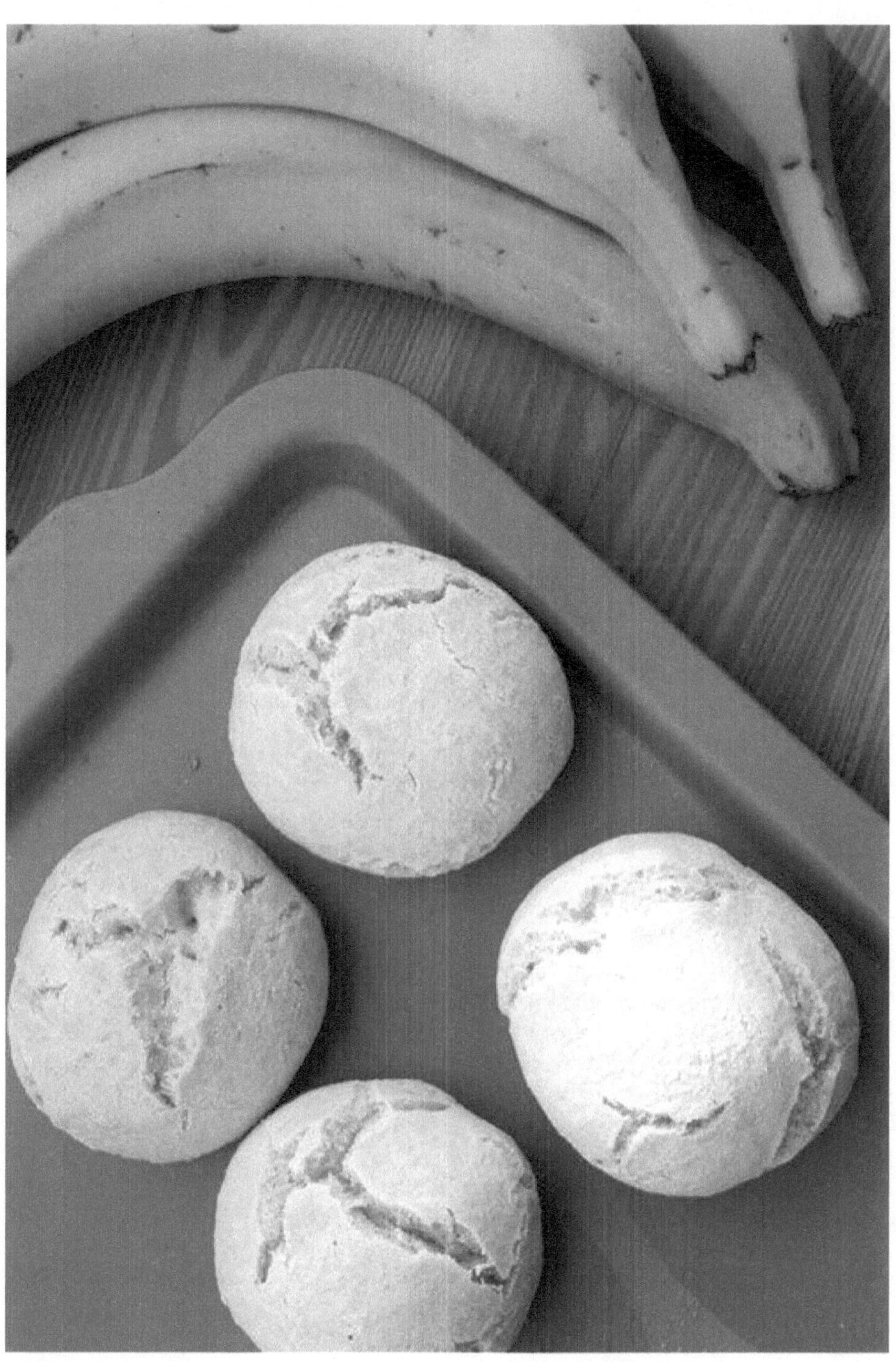

Soft and Fluffy Plantain Buns

Prep time: 15 minutes // Cook time: 15-20 minutes

Thanksgiving | Christmas | New Year | Easter

Course: Breakfast

Servings: 5 Servings

Calories: 175 kcal

These soft and fluffy plantain buns are as versatile as they are delicious. Enjoy with your favorite breakfast meat for a satisfying breakfast sandwich, stuffed with meats and veggies for a lunch sandwich, or as slider buns for supper! Get creative and enjoy the simplified egg-free baking method that is vegan as well as AIP and requires no gelatin!

Ingredients

- q1 green plantain, peeled and shredded (about 3/4 cup)
- q1 and 1/4 cup tapioca starch, plus 1-2 Tbsp extra if needed to dry dough
- q2 Tbsp coconut flour
- 1/8 tsp baking soda
- 1/4 tsp cream of tartar powder
- 1/4 tsp unrefined salt
- 1/2 cup coconut milk (Aroy-D has no added thickener or BPA)
- q2 Tbsp olive oil

optional: 1/2 to 1 Tbsp pressed or minced fresh garlic

Instructions

1. Preheat oven to 400 degrees Fahrenheit.
2. Peel the plantain using a sharp knife.
3. Cut off both tips then cut a slit down the length of the plantain peel (trying to only cut the peel and not the fruit). Lift and remove peel using fingers.
4. Cut multiple slits on 2-3 sides to make it easier. Using a hand grater or the grater attachment to your food processor, grate the peeled plantain. You should yield around 3/4 cup shreds.
5. In a large bowl combine tapioca starch, coconut flour, baking soda, cream of tartar, and salt and stir to combine well.
6. Then, add coconut milk, olive oil, and garlic (if using) and stir well to combine. Finally, add in the shredded plantain and use your hands to work it into a dough.

7   If dough is too wet, add 1-2 Tbsp tapioca starch. If it is too dry, add in coconut milk 1 Tbsp at a time.

8   Divide dough into 8 pieces and roll each into a ball. Place on a parchment paper-lined cookie sheet and bake for 15-20 min, until outsides are slightly golden.

9   Allow to cool several minutes before serving, and enjoy!

Apple Crisp

Prep time: 15 minutes // Cook time: 30-40 minutes

Thanksgiving | Christmas | New Year | Easter

Yield: 6 servings

A delicious Fall treat that's autoimmune paleo and allergy-friendly!

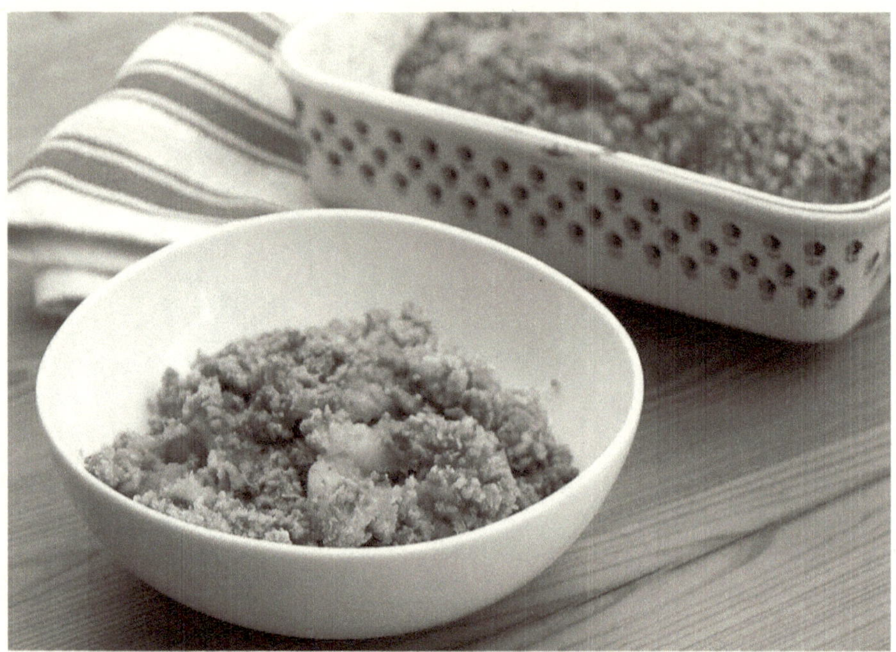

Ingredients

For the Filling

- 7-9 small Granny Smith apples (about 1.5 lbs), peeled, cored, and cut into wedges
- q1 tsp cinnamon
- juice of 1/2 lemon

For the Topping

- 3/4 cup shredded coconut (unsweetened)
- 1/3 cup coconut flour
- 1/3 cup sucanat
- 1/4 cup coconut oil, softened

- 1/4 cup coconut oil, softened or melted
- 3/4 tsp cinnamon powder (or, if tolerated, pumpkin pie spice blend)
- few pinches unrefined salt

Instructions

1. Preheat oven to 350 degrees Fahrenheit. If necessary, soften your coconut oil and coconut oil by placing the jars in a bowl filled with hot water for several minutes.
2. Peel and core the apples, then slice into about 6-8 wedges per apple. Place wedges in a medium/small baking dish -- I use a vintage dish that's about 2 quarts (it measures almost 11"x9").
3. If your baking dish is a lot larger, you will need to increase the amount of topping so that all the apples are covered.
4. If it's smaller, either decrease the amount of topping or you may need to increase the cooking time to compensate for a thicker topping layer.
5. Squeeze lemon juice and sprinkle cinnamon on top of the apple wedges and toss with a spoon to coat them evenly.
6. Add coconut shreds, coconut flour, sucanat, cinnamon powder (or pumpkin pie spice blend, if using), and unrefined salt to a mixing bowl and stir to combine evenly. I like to use my pastry blender to do this.
7. Add coconut butter and coconut oil to the dry ingredients and use the pastry blender to form the dough. Finish the dough with your hands, kneading it gently until it reaches a smooth consistency. It should be moist, yet crumbly. Add additional coconut oil if it feels too dry.
8. Crumble the topping on top of the apple wedges and use your fingers to press it down, forming a crust.
9. Bake at 350F until done, about 30-40 minutes. The topping should be golden brown.
10. Let cool about 5 minutes outside of the oven, then dig in and enjoy! If you have any leftovers, they keep well in the fridge in a covered container for several days. Just reheat for a few minutes in the oven when you're ready to eat them.

PUMPKIN FUDGE – DAIRY & EGG FREE, GAPS-FRIENDLY

Prep Time: 10 min//Cook Time: 5 min

Thanksgiving | Christmas

Gluten/Dairy/Egg/Nut-Free!

Category: Desserts

Allergen-free pumpkin fudge – a family favorite!

Ingredients

- 1/2 cup pumpkin puree, either homemade or canned will work (where to buy pumpkin puree)
- 1/3 cup coconut butter
- 3 tablespoons maple syrup – You can substitute with your preferred sweetener, but it will change the texture. You may also substitute with raw honey.
- 1/2 teaspoon vanilla
- 1/4 teaspoon cinnamon
- pinch ground ginger
- 1/8 tsp sea salt

Instructions

1. Combine all ingredients in a small pot or saucepan.
2. Heat on stove on the lowest setting, just enough to warm everything up. Stir constantly so you don't scorch the coconut butter.
3. You're not cooking it, just warming it up so the flavors will meld and it will spread a little easier. It should only take a minute for this to warm up. It will be quite thick and that's okay.
4. Pour into a small, flat container of your choice. I like using this to help spread it.
5. Place in fridge for at least 20 minutes to harden. And if you really can't wait, the freezer will do the job quicker – but the fridge keeps it at a more preferred temperature for cutting and serving.
6. If you do put it in the freezer, let it thaw a minute before serving.

NOTES

You could serve with powdered sugar sprinkled on top (If you are not on Sugar Free diet)

Pumpkin Spice Cake with Gingersnap Crust

Prep Time: 20 Mins // Cook Time: 30 Mins

Thanksgiving | Christmas

Serves: 6-8

Ingredients

For the Crust:

- ¾ cup arrowroot powder
- ¼ teaspoon sea salt
- 1½ cups dates, pitted and soaked in hot water for 5 minutes
- 2 tablespoons maple syrup
- 2 tablespoons lard (or coconut oil)
- 1½ teaspoons fresh grated ginger root

For the Filling:

- 3 cups pureed pumpkin
- ½ cup maple syrup
- ¼ cup lard (or coconut oil)
- 2½ tablespoons gelatin
- 1½ tablespoons cinnamon
- ¼ teaspoon ground cloves
- ¼ teaspoon sea salt

For the Frosting:

- ⅓ cup arrowroot powder
- 2½ tablespoons lard (or coconut oil)
- 2 tablespoons honey

Instructions

1. Preheat the oven to 325 degrees F and grease an 8-inch spring-form pan with either lard or coconut oil.
2. Drain the dates, and place all of the ingredients in a food processor and process for a minute, until a thick and sticky mixture forms.
3. You may be able to do this in a high-powered blender using the tamper, but be sure to stop to scrape the sides and take breaks because it will be hard on the motor.
4. Don't overmix here -- you want the dates to be slightly chunky and not completely incorporated.

5   Transfer the mixture to the spring-form pan and spread evenly along the bottom with a spatula. Bake in the oven for 18 to 20 minutes, or until a knife comes out clean when gently inserted. Set aside to cool.

6   Combine all of the filling ingredients, cold in a pot. Turn the heat on medium-low, and heat, stirring constantly, for 5 to 10 minutes.

7   The mixture should liquefy and the gelatin should dissolve. If you still have some chunks after 10 minutes, transfer to a blender and blend for a few seconds to incorporate.

8   Pour into the spring-form pan over the gingersnap crust. Place in the refrigerator to set for at least 3 hours.

9   To make the frosting, combine all of the ingredients in a small bowl. A thick, spreadable frosting should form.

10 If it is too runny, add more arrowroot, a teaspoon at a time until desired thickness is reached.

11 The frosting will harden when placed in the refrigerator and soften at room temperature (although it shouldn't melt).

12 When you are ready to frost your cake, you can either use a frosting kit or apply it to the top with a spatula.

NOTES

Note: Do not add fresh ginger to the filling ingredients -- it has an enzyme that breaks down the gelatin and will cause the cake not to set properly.

This cake freezes well -- if you don't eat it all, don't be afraid to freeze a few slices for later!

Paleo Marshmallows

Course: Dessert

Dairy Free, Gluten Free, Keto, Low Carb, Paleo

Thanksgiving | Christmas | New year| Birthday

Prep Time: 15 Minutes || Cook Time: 5 Minutes

Setting Time: 6 Hours

Servings: 25

Calories: 18 Kcal

Extra light, fluffy, chewy and just 3 ingredients! Yup, these sugar free, paleo and keto marshmallows are easy to whip up and a delight to devour. Think low carb s'mores in your foreseeable (i.e. immediate) future!

Ingredients

- 1/2 cup cold water
- 3 tablespoons gelatin preferably grass-fed
- 2/3 cup water
- 2/3-2 cups xylitol or allulose (we use 1 cup for xylitol & 1 1/3 cup for allulose)*
- 1/4 teaspoon kosher salt
- 2 teaspoons vanilla extract

SERVING SUGGESTIONS

- dark chocolate such as Lily's
- keto graham crackers
- raspberry chia jam

Instructions

1. Have all your ingredients handy, measured out, and make sure you won't be disturbed for 20 minutes. Seriously! They're easy and quick, but you need to work through the steps continuously and quickly.
2. Line a 9x9-inch pan with foil and grease well with coconut oil. Set aside. If using a stand mixer, fit it with the whisk attachment; otherwise have your hand mixer handy and ready to go.
3. Pour the cold water (1/2 cup) into your stand mixer's bowl or a large glass bowl. Sprinkle the gelatin in, mix thoroughly with a fork, and allow to bloom for 10 minutes while you melt the sweetener.

4. Pour the remaining water (2/3 cup) into a saucepan, and pour in the xylitol or allulose into the center without stirring (they don't form crystals, but just in case).

5. Bring to a boil over medium heat, allowing the sweetener to completely dissolve by giving the saucepan some light shakes, keeping the mixture at a rolling boil for about 2 minutes. If you've got a thermometer, temperature reaches about 210°F/100°C.

6. But don't worry if you don't have one; just be sure to let it boil for about 2 minutes to ensure maximum temperature is reached (sugar alcohols don't have the candy-making properties of sugar, so they don't heat up past a certain point).

7. You'll have to work quickly at this point to ensure no heat is lost. Turn on your mixer on low to break up the gelatin, and quickly pour in your hot syrup (trying to avoid the sides of your bowl so it doesn't cool down).

8. Increase your speed to high, and whisk non-stop for about 15 minutes. Sprinkle in the salt at about minute 8 and the vanilla extract at minute 12 (if you're adding stevia drops, do so at this point).

9. When ready, the mixture will be stiff and hold it's shape well, and if you're using a glass bowl it will feel only lightly warm to touch. The batter with xylitol won't be as fluffy as one with allulose, but it will still be light and stiff.

10. Turn mixer off, and quickly pour the marshmallow batter onto your prepared dish. Don't worry too much about what's left behind in the whisk etc, or your marshmallows will likely set in the bowl itself! Keep in mind that xylitol sets much quicker than allulose, so extra speed is required.

11. Allow your marshmallows to dry, uncovered and at room temperature, for 6 hours or preferably overnight. Gently remove from pan and cut with a greased knife. In my experience keto marshmallows don't need dusting as they're not overly sticky, and a touch of coconut oil does wonders if need be.

12. We did do a light dust of powdered sweetener as they were sticking to the counter while shooting (think summer heat)- so just store them in a cool, dry place for a couple weeks and in the freezer after.

RECIPE NOTES

Just note that erythritol in any shape and form isn't recommended (at all!) as crystalizes.

Keto Snickerdoodle Cookies

(Nut Free, Paleo)

Thanksgiving | Christmas | New Year | Easter |Birthday

Prep Time: 10 mins // Cook Time: 10

Yield: 18

Serving size: 1 cookie

Folks, it's a freaking Christmas miracle. I made a cookie without chocolate in it. Seriously. In general, when it comes to sweets I go chocolate or citrus... but snickerdoodle? Who am I even? Well, I am the wizard that came up with these delightful keto cookies

Cinnamon and sweet soft snickerdoodle cookies that are gluten free and low carb!

Ingredients

- 2 large eggs
- 1 teaspoon vanilla extract
- 1/3 cup + 2 tablespoons erythritol (maple or coconut sugar for paleo)
- ¼ cup (½ stick) coconut oil
- 1/3 cup + 1 teaspoon coconut flour
- ½ teaspoon baking soda
- Pinch of fine Himalayan salt
- 1 tablespoon gelatin or agar agar gum (optional)
- 2 tablespoons ceylon cinnamon
- 1/4 teaspoon nutmeg (optional)

Instructions

1. Preheat the oven to 350°F. Line a baking sheet with parchment paper.
2. In a large bowl, whisk the eggs until frothy with a fork or wire whisk. Add the vanilla extract, 1/3 cup granulated sweetener, and coconut oil and whisk until well combined.
3. Add the coconut flour, baking soda, gelatin, and salt to the wet ingredients. Using a rubber spatula, mix the ingredients together until a dough forms.
4. Using a 4CM cookie scoop or teaspoon make the cookies on the lined sheet pan.
5. The recipe makes 18. Using the palm of your hand, gently flatten the balls so they are about ½ inch thick.

6. Combine the cinnamon, nutmeg, and 2 tablespoons sweetener and dust the cookies with it. You can sprinkle it on or use a fine-mesh sieve to dust it on. Alternatively, you can roll the cookie balls in the cinnamon mix before putting them on the cookie sheet and flattening them.
7. Bake for 8-10 minutes, until the edges are lightly browned.
8. Remove from the oven and let the cookies cool to room temperature on the baking sheet before handling.
9. The more they cool, the chewier they will be. Store in an airtight container at room temperature for up to 5 days.

Calories: 44, Fat: 3g, Carbohydrates: 3g, Fiber: 1g, Protein: 2g

Pumpkin Cookies Recipe

Moderate Protein, Sugar- and Gluten-Free

Thanksgiving | Christmas

Prep Time: 15 mins // Cook Time: 30

Ingredients

- 2 Cups Almond Flour
- 1/2 Cup Pure Pumpkin
- 1 Large Egg
- 1/2 cup Coconut oil
- 1 tsp Pure Vanilla Extract
- 1/2 tsp Baking Powder
- 1/2 tsp Pumpkin Pie Spice
- 1 tsp Liquid Stevia OR 1/8 tsp Stevia Powder OR 1/2 cup Stevia in the Raw, Splenda, or other Sweetener

Instructions

1. Preheat oven to 300
2. Add all ingredients to a mixing bowl and mix until well combined.
3. Roll into 27 balls and place on a greased cookie sheet. Using a fork press dough down lightly.
4. Bake for 20-23 minutes.
5. Allow to cool for 5 minutes.

This is for 1 serving (1 cookie)

Calories: 82, Total Fat: 8g, Cholesterol: 16mg, Sodium: 34mg, Potassium: 66mg, Carbohydrates: 2g, Dietary Fiber = 1g, Net Carbs= 1g, Dietary Fiber 1g, Sugars: 0g, Protein: 2g

Chocolate Silk Pie

Prep Time: 15 mins // Cook Time: 1 hour

Thanksgiving | Christmas | New Year | Easter

Yields: 10 servings of Chocolate Silk Pie

The crust of this pie is a simple almond flour crust. This flaky, slightly

sweet, pastry dough provides a lovely contrast from the sweeter silky chocolate filling. The crust is baked prior to filling since the filling does not required baking.

The luscious filling has a cream cheese base with rich cocoa. There's an additional hint of coconut oil for added richness. Whipped cream is folded in to lighten it and provide a silky, velvety, texture.

This chocolate silk pie will satisfy any dessert craving you might have. With this recipe, you can curb that chocolate dessert craving without the guilt!

Ingredients

For the crust:

- 1 ½ cups almond flour
- ½ teaspoon baking powder
- 1/8 teaspoon. salt
- 1/3 cup granulated stevia/erythritol blend
- 3 tablespoons coconut oil
- 1 medium egg
- 1 ½ teaspoons vanilla extract
- 1 teaspoon coconut oil, for greasing the pan

For the filling:

- 16 ounces **Paleo cream cheese**, room temperature
- 4 tablespoons sour cream
- 4 tablespoons coconut oil
- 1 tablespoon vanilla extract
- ½ cup granulated stevia/erythritol blend
- ½ cup cocoa powder
- 1 cup whipping cream
- 2 teaspoons granulated stevia/erythritol blend, for whipped cream
- 1 teaspoon vanilla extract, for whipped cream

Instructions

1. Preheat oven to 375 degrees Fahrenheit. Generously butter a 9" pie pan with 1 tsp. coconut oil
2. In a medium mixing bowl, combine almond flour, baking powder, salt and 1/3 cup stevia/erythritol blend. Using a whisk, blend the dry ingredients together.
3. Add coconut oil to dry ingredients. Using a pastry blender, whisk or a fork, cut the coconut oil into dry ingredients until the mixture forms into coarse crumbs.
4. Add egg and vanilla extract and stir until the dough forms into a ball.
5. Transfer the dough to the prepared pan and spread out the dough using your fingers until it evenly covers the bottom and sides of the pan.
6. Wetting your hands with cold water can help prevent the dough from sticking to your fingers. Flute edges if desired.
7. Using a fork, poke holes in the bottom and sides of crust to prevent bubbles from forming as it bakes.
8. Place crust in the oven and bake for 11 minutes. Remove crust from the oven and loosely cover edges with foil. Return it to oven for 5 to 8 more minutes or until the bottom of the crust is golden brown. Allow the crust to cool completely before filling
9. To prepare the filling, place cream cheese, sour cream, coconut oil, vanilla extract, ½ cup stevia/erythritol blend and cocoa powder in a medium bowl.
1. Using a mixer on low speed, blend ingredients to combine, then increase to high speed and beat until fluffy.
2. Place the whipping cream in a separate small bowl. Using clean mixer beaters, whip the cream on high speed until soft peaks for. Add the 2 tsp. sweetener and 1 tsp. vanilla extract and beat until stiff peaks form.
3. Gently fold 1/3 of the whipped cream mixture into the cream cheese mixture to lighten. Add remaining whipped cream mixture and fold it in gently. The idea is to blend the two mixtures together without breaking the bubbles in the cream.
4. Scoop the filling into the crust and smooth the top with a spoon. Cover and refrigerate your keto chocolate silk pie for at least 3 hours before serving.

Each serving comes out to be 448.7 Calories, 43.59g Fats, 5.88g Net Carbs, and 9.48g Protein.

Chicken fried Steak with Creamy Sausage gravy

Thanksgiving | Christmas | New Year | Easter

Yield: 4 Servings 1x

Ingredients

FOR THE CHICKEN FRIED STEAK

- 1 lb cube steak, 4 pieces pounded 1/4 inch thick
- Sea salt and black pepper
- 1/4 cup Paleo heavy cream
- 2 large eggs
- 1 1/2 cups crushed pork rinds
- 1/2 cup vegan Parmesan cheese, grated
- 1 1/2 tsp onion powder
- 1 1/2 tsp garlic powder
- 1 tsp paprika
- Pinch of cayenne pepper
- Cooking oil

FOR THE CREAMY SAUSAGE GRAVY

- 2 tbsp coconut oil
- 12 oz pork breakfast sausage links (I like to use maple sausage links)
- 2/3 cup onion, diced
- 3 cloves garlic, minced
- 11/2 cups Paleo heavy cream
- 1 tbsp fresh parsley, chopped
- 1/2 tsp sea salt

Instructions

FOR THE CHICKEN FRIED STEAK

1. Sprinkle the cube steaks with sea salt and black pepper on both sides.
2. In a shallow bowl, combine the heavy cream and eggs. Fork whisk.
3. Combine the pork rinds, Parmesan cheese, onion powder, garlic powder, paprika and cayenne pepper. Pour the mixture into a thin layer on a large plate. This will be your breading.
4. In a large cast-iron skillet over medium-high heat, heat 1/4 to 1/2 inch of oil.

5. Dip the cube steak into the egg wash and then dredge in the "breading," coating thoroughly on both sides.
6. Drop the breaded cube steak into the oil. Fry until crispy and golden brown, about 3 minutes for each side.
7. Top with the Creamy Sausage Gravy.

FOR THE CREAMY SAUSAGE GRAVY

1. Heat the coconut oil in a large skillet over medium heat. Once the ghee is melted, add
2. the sausage (crumbled if ground, sliced if using link sausage). Cook until the sausage is browned. Using a slotted spoon, remove the sausage from the pan, retaining the drippings. Set the sausage aside.
3. To the drippings in the pan, add the onion and garlic. Lower the heat to medium-low and cook until the onion is translucent and soft. Stir often to avoid burning the garlic.
4. To the pan, add the heavy cream, parsley and sea salt. Increase the heat to medium and bring to a boil. Once the gravy begins to boil, lower the heat to low and simmer. Once the gravy begins to thicken, add the sausage back to the pan.
5. Pour the gravy over top of the Chicken Fried Steak and ENJOY!

Calories: 676, Fat: 51g, Protein: 47g, Net Carbohydrate: 5g

Savory Breakfast Cookies

Prep time: 15 minutes || Cook time: 40-45 minutes

Thanksgiving | Christmas | New Year | Easter

Yield: 12

Ingredients

- 1/2 cup coconut flour
- 1/2 tsp baking soda
- 1/2 tsp unrefined salt
- 1 tsp dried rosemary
- 1 tsp dried granulated garlic
- 4 Tbsp. extra-virgin olive oil
- 6 Tbsp. coconut oil
- 4 Tbsp. gelatin (Great Lakes brand is from grass-fed cows) **NOTE: Do NOT use the green "collagen hydrolysate" -- it won't work!
- 1 cup room temperature filtered water
- 1/2 Tbsp. raw apple cider vinegar
- parchment paper

Instructions

1. Preheat oven to 350F.
2. Prepare your gelatin for use. First, you will have to "bloom" it, then you will melt it. Add water to a small pot and sprinkle/rain gelatin on top, about 1/2 Tbsp. at a time in a single layer. Do NOT let it clump or pour it all in one place.
3. You want to spread it out evenly. If not, clumps may form that are difficult to dissolve and the texture in the final product will be negatively affected.
4. Be patient with this part! I use a whisk and vigorously stir the gelatin after each 1/2 Tbsp. has been added and wetted.
5. Once all gelatin has been wetted, heat over medium low for several minutes until all gelatin has melted and you have a translucent liquid. Stir occasionally with your whisk until dissolved.
6. While you are waiting on the gelatin to melt, mix all dry ingredients together in a large bowl. (I recommend sifting the coconut flour to remove any clumps. Be sure to evenly distribute the baking soda throughout.)
7. Once gelatin is completely dissolved, add remaining wet ingredients to gelatin (oils and apple cider vinegar), then pour all wet ingredients into the bowl with your dry ingredients and stir with a large spoon.

8. At first, the batter will seem like it is going to be too runny, but as you stir it the batter will thicken up and soon look like a normal batter.

9. Use your spoon to divide batter into 12 cookies/biscuits onto a parchment paper-lined baking sheet (trust me -- do NOT skip the parchment paper!) Bake at 350F for about 40-45 minutes, or until the cookies are golden and the edges are slightly browned and you can easily lift them with a spatula.

10. If they stick to the paper or come apart in the middle, they are not ready yet. For some reason, the gelatin makes these have a longer cooking time than they would have if made with eggs.

11. Serve immediately and enjoy! Store leftovers in an air-tight container and reheat in the oven for several minutes before serving. I do not recommend eating them cold as they do not have a great texture. They will be crispier the second time they are heated, too.

NOTE: Be sure to wash your pot, whisk, bowl, spoon, and anything else that touched the gelatin right away. If you let it sit, the gelatin will harden and become much harder to clean!

Garlic Bacon Roasted Cauliflower with Herbed Aioli

Serves: 6

Prep Time: 10 mins || Cook Time: 30 min

Thanksgiving | Christmas | New Year | Easter

Cooking Type: Roasting

Course: Main dish

This roasted cauliflower is packed with goodies like crispy savory bacon, garlic, and served with a creamy herbed aioli for dipping. It's paleo, Whole foods compliant and keto friendly. Perfect as a holiday side dish or for anytime!

Ingredients

- 1 head cauliflower cut into florets
- slices nitrate free bacon sugar free for Whole foods
- cloves garlic minced
- tsp rosemary fresh, minced
- Sea salt and pepper to taste

aioli:

- 1/2 cup homemade mayo*
- cloves garlic minced
- 1/2 tsp fresh lemon juice
- 1 tsp minced fresh herbs I used sage, rosemary and thyme
- Sea salt and black pepper to taste

Instructions

1. Preheat your oven to 425 degrees. Spread cauliflower florets in a single layer on a large baking sheet. Cut bacon into pieces, then sprinkle all over cauliflower.
2. Roast in the preheated oven for 15 mins, then stir and return to single layer. Continue to roast another 5 mins or until bacon is mostly crisp, then, sprinkle with the garlic and rosemary.
3. Continue to roast another 5-7 mins or until all is toasty. Once done, sprinkle with sea salt and pepper to taste (remember the bacon adds salt, so be careful!)
4. During the last 5-7 mins of roasting, whisk together all aioli ingredients in a small bowl. Serve alongside the cauliflower for dipping. Enjoy!

*You can also use a paleo store bought Mayo version, but I highly recommend starting with my easy homemade recipe for the best flavor.

Calories: 230kcalFat: 22gSaturated fat: 5gCholesterol: 22mgSodium: 270mgPotassium: 112mgCarbohydrates: 2gProtein: 3gVitamin A: 25%Vitamin C: 10.2%Calcium: 16%Iron: 0.4%

Keto Teriyaki Bowl

Prep Time: 10 Mins // Cook Time: 35 Mins

Thanksgiving | Christmas | New Year | Easter

Yield: 4

Serving Size: 1/4 of Recipe

Recipe Type: Main dish

Ingredients

MEATBALLS

- 2 pounds ground beef 85%lean
- 1inch nub fresh ginger, peeled and zested
- 1 heaping teaspoon grated citrus zest (I used orange and lime)
- 2 teaspoons garlic powder
- 2 teaspoon fine salt
- 1 teaspoon dried parsley
- 2 tablespoons minced fresh cilantro, more to garnish
- Half a ripe hass avocado

FOR COOKING

- 4 tablespoons avocado oil, more as needed

SAUCE

- 1/3 cup bone broth
- 1 tablespoon fish sauce
- 1 tablespoon red wine vinegar
- ¼ cup coconut aminos, divided
- 1 scoop gelatin

FIXINGS

- 4 cups shredded Brussels sprouts
- 5 cloves garlic sliced

- 4 large eggs

NOODLES

- 4 bags shirataki noodles or veggie noodles like zoodles for Whole foods

Instructions

1. Pre-heat oven to 400F.
2. In a large bowl mix together, the ground beef with the rest of the meatball ingredients until well combined, the avocado should be completely mixed in with only traces of green specks in the meat, no chunks left. Shape 12 large meatballs.
3. Bring a small sauce pot full of water to a boil. Put the 4 large eggs, gently in the pot. Boil for 7 minutes, then drain the water and add ice to the eggs, set aside.
4. Toss the Brussels sprouts on a sheet pan with 2 tablespoons avocado oil and 1 teaspoon salt. Spread them out flat over the sheet pan and pop in the oven- middle rack.
5. Heat a large skillet over medium heat. When it comes to temperature add 2 tablespoons of avocado oil to the skillet and brown 6 meatballs at a time, 2 minutes a side, then transfer to a sheet pan. Repeat with the remaining meatballs and then put them in the oven.
6. Add the meatballs to the oven, with the Brussels sprouts, for 10-15 minutes until the sauce and noodles are ready.
7. In the same sauce pot where you boiled the eggs heat the bone broth with the fish sauce, red wine vinegar, and 2 tablespoons coconut aminos. Bring to a boil and reduce for 10 minutes.
8. Add 1 scoop gelatin to the remaining coconut aminos and let it sit until it gels up solid.
9. In the meantime, drain and rinse your noodles and submerge in cool water. Set aside.

10. Heat the skillet where the meatballs were browned and add a little extra avocado oil. Then add in the sliced garlic and fry until golden. Remove from the skillet.

11. Drain the noodles, add to the skillet, sprinkle with salt and sauté in the garlic infused fat for a few minutes while you finish the sauce. They will coat in the fat and get brown and yummy!

12. Remove the bone broth reduction from the heat, scoop in the solid coconut amino-gelatin mass and whisk into broth until smooth and thick. Set aside.

13. Remove the toasty Brussels sprouts and cooked meatballs from the oven.

14. Assemble your bowls.

15. Divide the noodles in between 4 large bowls, then the Brussels sprouts. Add 3 meatballs to each bowl. Garnish with fried garlic, minced cilantro. Peel the eggs and halve them. Add ½ -1 egg to each bowl.

16. Spoon thick teriyaki sauce generously over each bowl and dig in!!

Recipe Notes:

The Macros Include ALL THE MEATBALLS AND ALL THE SAUCE. The recipe is best with 3 meatballs per person. There will be leftover meat and leftover sauce. However, if you divide the entire recipe by 4... the macros are as listed.

CALORIES: 821, FAT: 56g, CARBOHYDRATES: 18g, FIBER: 7.8g, PROTEIN: 53g

Breakfast Sausage

Serves: 12

Thanksgiving | Christmas | New Year | Easter

Prep Time: 5 mins || Cook Time: 10 min

Cooking Type: Baking

Course: Breakfast

Whole foods Breakfast Sausage (Whole and Paleo) - clean eating is simple with this easy homemade breakfast sausage recipe. Great for freezing too!

Ingredients

- 1 lb ground turkey (or pork or chicken)
- 1 teaspoon Italian seasoning
- 1 teaspoon sage
- 1/2 teaspoon all-purpose salt free blend
- 1/2 teaspoon sea salt
- cooking oil of choice

Instructions

1. Combine ground turkey and seasonings in a bowl. Mix well with your hands and form 12 patties.
2. Heat a large skillet over medium heat. Add cooking oil (avocado, coconut, or olive oil) or ghee to the pan. Add patties to the pan (in batches) and cook 3-4 minutes per side, until nicely browned and cooked through.
3. Remove from pan and drain on paper towels if desired. Serve immediately, refrigerate, or freeze for future use.

Alternative to patties, make ground sausage by cooking ground turkey and spices together in the oil, breaking up into pieces.

Calories: 68kcal | Protein: 7g | Fat: 4g | Saturated Fat: 1g | Cholesterol: 31mg | Sodium: 123mg | Potassium: 80mg | Vitamin A: 30IU | Calcium: 11mg | Iron: 0.5mg

Pizza Breakfast Casserole

Prep Time: 10 Mins // Cook Time: 35 Mins

Thanksgiving | Christmas | New Year

Yield: 8

Recipe Type: Breakfast

An easy make-ahead breakfast bake with all the Italian flavors of your favorite pizza!

Ingredients

- 2 tbsp olive oil
- 12 eggs
- 2 tsp Italian seasoning
- 1 tsp sea salt
- 1/2 onion diced
- 1 green pepper diced
- 1 red pepper diced
- 1 lb Ground Italian or Breakfast Sausage if not using turkey sausage, sugar and nitrate free brand
- 10-12 regular or turkey pepperoni, sugar and nitrate free brand
- 1 14.5 can diced tomatoes drained
- Turkey Sausage
- 1 lb lean ground turkey
- 1 tsp fennel seed
- 1 tsp salt
- 2 tsp sage
- 1 tsp thyme
- 1 tsp black pepper
- 1/2 tsp cayenne
- 1/2 tsp garlic powder

Instructions

1. Preheat oven to 350. Spray a 9x13 inch casserole dish with olive oil or avocado oil.
2. Make sausage. Heat a large sauté pan over medium high heat and add 1 tbsp olive oil. If making turkey sausage, add all ingredients and cook 5-7 minutes until no longer pink.
3. If using other sausage, cook 5-7 minutes until browned and cooked through.

4. Add cooked sausage to the bottom of the casserole dish. Using the same pan, add remaining olive oil and chopped onions and peppers.
5. Cook until onion is opaque and beginning to soften, 3-4 minutes. Add onions and peppers to the casserole dish along with the drained canned diced tomatoes.
6. Whisk 12 eggs with the Italian seasoning in a bowl. Pour the eggs over the meat and veggies and stir to combine. Top with pepperonis.
7. Bake for 25-30 minutes until cooked through and the eggs are firm/set. Top with ranch dressing and enjoy! Store in the fridge for up to 5 days.

Veggie Keto Burgers

Prep Time: 15 Mins // Cook Time: 35 Mins

Thanksgiving | Christmas | New Year

Servings: 6

These are so delicious and super easy to do! I make a huge batch and I freeze them individually in zip lock bags. If you want one or two because they are that GOOD and TASTY you can either toast **them or bake in oven.**

Ingredients:

- Optional: Spaghetti Squash or Sweet potatoes 1 Cup - Optional
- 4 Tbl Psyllium Husk Powder
- 1 Cup Chopped Parsley
- 1 Cup Chopped Cilantro
- 1 Cup chopped Kale
- 2 Cups Green Pea
- 2 Large Yellow or White Onions
- 3 Cups Zucchini
- 1 Cup Sun Dried Tomatoes
- 1/2 Cup Mushrooms
- 1 Cup Peppers
- 10 Cloves Garlic
- 3 Whole Lemons
- 2 Tbl Pink Salt
- 1 Tbl Black pepper
- 2 Tbl Paprika
- 3 Tbl Oregano
- 1 Tbl Dried Dill
- 1 Tbl Mustard
- 1/2 Cup Grape seed Oil or Olive Oil

Instructions:

1. Stir Fry everything together.
2. Add more or less spice as you like.
3. Blend everything together except for the Green Pea.
4. Mix everything well.
5. Form into Shapes
6. Bake on 375F for 12-15 minutes
7. Let cool them pack and store in Freezer.
8. Enjoy!

Low Carb Blueberry Muffins

Prep Time: 10 Mins // Cook Time: 30 Mins

Thanksgiving | Christmas | New Year

Yield: 12

Serving Size: 1 Muffin

Ingredients

- 1/2 cup coconut flour
- 6 tablespoons psyllium husk
- 1 teaspoon baking powder
- 1/2 teaspoon salt
- 1/2 cup unsweetened sunflower seed butter
- 1/4 cup softened coconut oil, ghee or tallow
- 4 large eggs, room temperature
- 3 tablespoons yacon syrup or 1/3 cup honest syrup
- 1/2 cup non-dairy milk of choice
- 1 teaspoon vanilla extract
- 2 tsp. lemon zest
- 1 cup blueberries

Instructions

1. Preheat oven to 350F. Line a muffin tin with cupcake liners.
2. In a large bowl whisk together the coconut flour, psyllium husk, baking powder and salt.
3. In a separate bowl beat together the sunflower seed butter, coconut oil, eggs, syrup, vanilla and milk until well combined and creamy.
4. Add the wet mix to the dry mix and beat until a dough forms.
5. Add in the blueberries and lemon zest and use a spatula to fold in.
6. Use a ¼ cup scoop per muffin. Bake in the center rack for 25- 30 minutes or until the muffins have risen, round and golden on top.

7. Coconut Flour Blueberry Muffins (paleo, keto, dairy free, nut free)

8. Remove from the oven and let cool. Store in an airtight container at room temperature for up to 5 days.

Recipe Notes:

You can also use Zero Syrup which is vegetable glycerin (a sugar alcohol) and monk fruit or Honest Syrup made of vegetable fiber and monk fruit. While the latter is free of sugar alcohols which is ideal for some, it is high very high in total carbs (fiber). Use 1/4 to 1/3 cup in this recipe instead of Yacon Syrup.

Calories: 176.2, Fat: 12.7g, Carbohydrates: 10.4g, Fiber: 6.5g, Protein: 5.2g

Gluten Free Pumpkin Bread Recipe

Prep Time 15 minutes // Cook Time 50 minutes

Thanksgiving | Christmas | Birthday

Servings 12

Calories 169kcal

A gluten free pumpkin bread recipe made with coconut flour with a taste and texture like the real thing, except it's low carb and completely sugar-free!

Ingredients

- 3/4 cup coconut flour
- 1/2 cup Sukrin Gold packed (or my brown sugar substitute)*
- 3 tbsp whey protein isolate
- 2 1/2 tsp baking powder
- 2 tsp cinnamon
- 1/2 tsp salt
- 6 large eggs
- 4 oz ghee, melted
- 2 tsp vanilla extract
- 1 tsp Stevia Glycerite
- 1 1/2 cup fresh, grated pumpkin (6 oz)

Topping (optional)

- 2 tbsp chopped pecans
- 2 tbsp Sukrin Gold

Instructions

1. Preheat the oven to 350 degrees F and place rack into the middle of the oven. Spray an 8x4 inch loaf pan with baking spray and cut a piece of parchment to fit inside and hand over the sides of the pan (see picture).
2. Pumpkin bread made with coconut flour in a pan with pumpkins and blue napkin.
3. Thoroughly mix the dry ingredients in a medium bowl.
4. Add the wet ingredients and grated pumpkin.
5. Blend with a hand mixer until fully incorporated and spoon into the prepared baking pan. Lift the pan a few inches above the counter and let it fall, knocking out any big air bubbles. Do this 2-3 times.
6. Sprinkle chopped pecans over the top of the bread and gently press into the batter. Sprinkle with the brown sugar substitute.

7. Bake for 50-60 minutes or until a toothpick inserted in the middle comes out clean, but the bread still sounds moist. Let cool in the pan for 5 minutes. Loosen the bread from the ends of the pan and lift the loaf to a cooling rack. Let cool completely.
8. Store in the refrigerator in a plastic bag for up to a week or freeze. Serves 12.

Calories: 169kcal | Carbohydrates: 5g | Protein: 7g | Fat: 13g | Sodium: 227mg | Fiber: 2g

Blackberry Coconut Fat Bombs

Prep Time 5 minutes // Cook Time 5 minutes

Thanksgiving | Christmas

Servings 16 small squares

Calories 170kcal

These sugar free blackberry coconut fat bombs are low carb and Paleo. Eat them between meals to stay in ketosis on a ketogenic diet during weight loss.

Ingredients

- 1 cup coconut butter see note for how to make homemade
- 1 cup coconut oil
- 1/2 cup fresh or frozen blackberries can use raspberries or strawberries if desired
- 1/2 teaspoon SweetLeaf stevia drops add a bit more for sweeter taste
- 1/4 teaspoon vanilla powder or 1/2 teaspoon vanilla extract
- 1 tablespoon lemon juice

Instructions

1. Place coconut butter, coconut oil and blackberries (if frozen) in a pot and heat over medium heat just until well combined.
2. In a food processor or small blender, add coconut oil mix and remaining ingredients. Process until smooth. NOTE: Separation may occur if coconut oil mixture is too hot. If using fresh berries, there is no need to cook them with the coconut oil and butter.
3. Spread out into a small pan lined with parchment paper (I used 6x6-inch container)
4. Refrigerate one hour or until mix has hardened.
5. Remove from container and cut into squares.
6. Store covered in the refrigerator.

Notes

- To make coconut butter, place about 2 cups unsweetened dried coconut flakes into food processor and process until butter forms (about 7-8 minutes) 0.8g net carbs
- The amount of berries can be increased for a sweeter and more intense berry taste.

Calories 170 Calories from Fat 168, Total Fat 18.7g 29%|Total Carbohydrates 3g 1%|Dietary Fiber 2.3g 9%|Protein 1.1g 2% |Net Carbs 0.7g| Carbs: 1.6%|Protein: 2.5%

Coconut Lemon Curd Cake

Prep Time: 1 hr 30 mins // Cook Time: 50 mins

Thanksgiving | Christmas | New Year | Birthday

Calories: 359 kcal

Servings: 12

A scrumptious and low carb coconut cake filled with a tangy sugar free lemon curd. The lemon curd and cake can be prepared several days in advance and refrigerated. Assemble and frost the cake the day before needed so the lemon curd will have time to set up.

Ingredients

Lemon Curd:

- 1/2 cup fresh lemon juice
- 1/2 cup granular Swerve Sweetener
- 3 large eggs
- 3 large egg yolks
- 3 tbsp. coconut oil
- 2 tsp arrowroot powder or cornstarch
- Zest from the lemons

Coconut Cake:

- 4 oz unsalted coconut oil softened
- 4 oz Paleo cream cheese softened
- 1/2 cup granular Swerve Sweetener
- 1 tsp coconut extract
- 1/2 tsp vanilla extract
- 1 cup almond flour
- 1 cup coconut flour
- 2 tsp baking powder
- 1/2 tsp salt
- 1/4 tsp xanthan gum
- 4 large eggs cold
- 3 large egg whites cold
- 2/3 cup almond milk cold

Whipped Cream Frosting:

- 1 1/3 cup heavy Coconut whipping cream
- 1/3 cup confectioners Swerve Sweetener

- 1/2 tsp vanilla extract
- 1 tsp coconut extract
- 1/8 tsp xanthan gum

Garnish:

- 1/2 cup flaked coconut for the outside of the cake

Raspberries optional

Instructions

Lemon Curd:

1. Mix the Swerve and arrowroot powder together in a small pot.
2. Add the egg yolks and lemon zest, whole eggs, and lemon juice whisking thoroughly between each addition.
3. Turn the heat to medium and whisk until the mixture just begins to thicken. Adjust the heat to medium-low and whisk briskly until the mixture thickens, all at once.
4. Turn off the heat and continue whisking for 1 minute. Whisk in the ghee. Strain the mixture into a clean bowl. Cool, cover with cling film and refrigerate overnight or up to 4 days.

Cake:

1. Preheat oven to 350 degrees F and position rack to the lower third. Spray two 6 x 2 -inch round pans (or three 8x1-inch pans) with baking spray and line the bottoms with parchment.
2. Add the first 5 ingredients to a medium bowl and cream until light and fluffy. Add the egg whites and beat again until light and fluffy. In a small bowl, add the remaining dry cake ingredients and whisk to combine and break up any lumps. Add 1/3 of the dry ingredients and beat until incorporated.
3. Add two eggs and beat until light and fluffy. Scrape down the bowl and repeat the procedure ending with the final addition of the dry ingredients. Lastly, add the almond milk and beat, keeping a nice fluffy texture.
4. Divide the batter between the prepared pans and spread with an offset spatula. Lift the pans a few inches off of the counter and drop 2-3 times to knock out any large air bubbles.
5. Place pans in the oven and raise the temperature to 400 degrees F for 10 minutes, then back to 350 degrees for 20-30 minutes more. The cakes are done when firm to the touch but they still sound a little moist. (Cooking time will be less with three 8-inch pans.)

Remove cakes from the oven and cover with a clean tea towel to cool completely.

6. They will sink a bit in the middle. Wrap with cling film and refrigerate until needed.

To Assemble:

1. Whip the heavy whipping cream with the sweetener and flavorings until almost stiff. Sprinkle the xanthan gum over the whipped cream and whip until very stiff and almost clumpy. Put 1/3 of the whipped cream into a pint ziploc bag and snip off 3/8 inch off the corner (or slide a large round open tip into the bag).
2. Remove and reserve 1/4 cup of lemon curd. Mix the remaining lemon curd to loosen it.
3. For 6-inch pans: Slightly slice off the tops to even out the cakes and then slice each cake in half horizontally. Place one cake half on the serving plate and squeeze a ring or dam of whipped cream along the inside edge of the cake. Spread 1/3 of the lemon curd on the cake up to the dam. Top with another layer of cake, pressing lightly to level. Follow the same procedure and repeat. Top with the remaining cake layer.
4. For 8-inch pans: Do the same as above except don't slice the cakes in half. Spread 1/2 of the lemon curd on the bottom cake layer up to the whipped cream dam. Top with another layer of cake and follow the same procedure. Top with the remaining cake layer.

To Decorate:

1. Frost the cake with the whipped cream. Using small handfuls, apply the flaked coconut to the sides of the cake. Stick 4-5 toothpicks into the top and carefully cover the cake in cling film. Refrigerate overnight.
2. Before serving, remove the toothpicks and mix the remaining lemon curd with enough water (2-3 tbsp.) to make a spoonable (but not runny) mixture. Spoon the lemon curd around the top edge of the cake, encouraging it to drip down. Spoon the rest of the lemon curd over the top of the cake and spread gently with the spoon or an offset spatula. Cut and serve.
3. NOTE: This cake is not overly sweet. If you like your desserts sweet, add liquid stevia drops or stevia glycerite to taste. Fresh raspberries make the perfect garnish.

Recipe Notes

Calories: 359, Fat: 32, Carbohydrates: 9, Fiber: 4, Protein: 9, NET CARBS: 4

Nut-free cheesecake

Prep Time: 30 minutes // Cook Time: 1 hour, 25 minutes

Thanksgiving | Christmas | New Year | Birthday

Category: Dessert

Yield: 12 slices

Serving Size: 1 slice

Calories Per Serving: 341

For Nut Allergy only

If have you been searching for keto nut free recipes This is the perfect keto nut free cheesecake recipe for you!

Ingredients

Crust:

- 1 cup (144g) sesame seeds
- ¾ cup (60g) unsweetened shredded coconut
- ¼ cup (2 oz) unsalted melted ghee
- 3 tbsp (36g) classic monk fruit sweetener
- 1 tsp cinnamon
- ⅛ tsp salt

Cheesecake Layer:

- 1 cup (192g) classic monk fruit sweetener
- 24 oz Paleo cream cheese, softened
- ¼ cup (60g) sour cream
- 1 tsp (5mL) lemon juice
- 1 tsp pure vanilla extract
- 3 eggs
- 1 egg yolk

Instructions

Crust:

1. Preheat oven to 300 degrees. Liberally coat bottom and sides of 9-inch springform pan with nonstick cooking spray.
2. Wrap bottom and sides of outside of pan with aluminum foil (this will ensure liquid from the water bath does not seep into the cheesecake when baking). Set aside.

3. In a food processor, pulse sesame seeds and shredded coconut until ground. Transfer mixture to mixing bowl and add melted ghee, monk fruit sweetener, cinnamon, and salt and mix with a fork until well-incorporated.
4. Spoon crust mixture into prepared springform pan and transfer pan to the oven to bake until the edges are golden brown, about 15 minutes.
5. After baking, remove pan from oven and allow to cool while preparing the cheesecake layer.

Cheesecake Layer:

1. In a food processor, pulse monk fruit sweetener until powdered. Transfer powdered monk fruit sweetener to mixing bowl and add cream cheese and sour cream and, using an electric mixer at medium-low speed, mix ingredients together until creamy and all cream cheese lumps are gone (a few small lumps are fine, but we just want to be sure all of the large lumps are mixed).
2. Using a rubber spatula, scrape sides and bottom of bowl to unsecure any cream cheese that has stuck to the bowl. Mix again. Add lemon juice and vanilla extract and mix again.

One at a time, add eggs and egg yolk and mix on medium-low speed until each egg is just barely mixed in. It's important to not over mix the eggs, otherwise the cheesecake surface may crack while baking.

3. Place foil-lined springform pan in center of large baking sheet. Pour enough water into baking sheet to fill ~1 inch of water.
4. Final Steps: Pour cream cheese mixture atop crust in springform pan. Return pan set in water bath to oven and bake until the center is almost set, but still "jiggly," about 1 hour, 10 minutes. Turn oven off and, using a wooden spoon, crack oven door open just slightly. Allow pan to sit in cooling oven for 1 hour.
5. Remove baking sheet with water bath and pan from oven. Remove pan from water bath. Remove and discard foil from outside of pan. Slide a knife around the edge of the cheesecake, to separate the edge of the cake from the pan. Transfer pan to refrigerator to chill uncovered for 4 hours, preferably overnight, before cutting and serving.

47%Total Fat 30.3g, 8%Total Carbohydrate 24.6g, 83%Dietary Fiber 20.7g, 17%Protein 8.6g

vegan bread rolls

Prep Time: 15 minutes // Cook Time: 1 hour

Thanksgiving | Christmas | New Year | Easter

Yield: 6 rolls

Category: Bread

Method: Bake

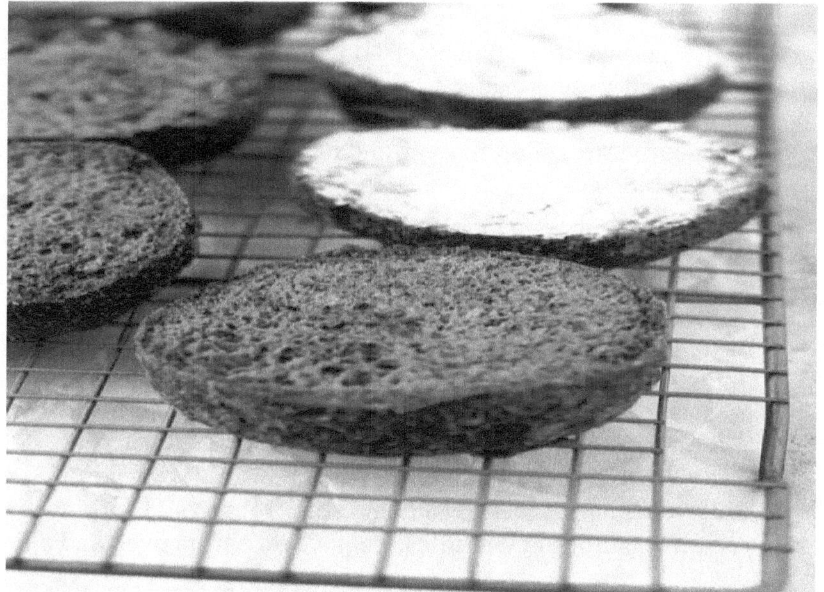

These Vegan Keto Bread Rolls are the most delicious, low-carb, and allergy-friendly way to enjoy bread! They can be topped with your favorite spread or cut in half and used as a bun!

This recipe is keto, low-carb, paleo, dairy-free, egg-free, gluten-free, grain-free, vegetarian, vegan, refined-sugar-free, and has only 3.3g net carbs per roll!

Ingredients

- Flax Egg
- 3 tbsp ground flax seeds
- 1/2 cup + 1 tbsp water

Bread Roll Dough

- 1 1/4 cup almond flour
- 1/3 cup ground flax seeds

* 1/2 cup psyllium husk powder
* 1 tsp salt
* 2 1/2 tsp baking soda
* 1 1/4 tsp cream of tartar
* 1 1/4 cup water

Instructions

1. Preheat oven to 375 degrees and line baking sheet with parchment paper.
2. For the flax egg, to a small bowl, add flax seeds and water and whisk together. Allow soaking for 5 minutes.
3. In a medium bowl, add dry ingredients and whisk together until fully incorporated. Add flax egg and mix with an electric mixer until well-combined.
4. In a small pot, bring water to boil.
5. With the electric mixer turned on, slowly pour boiling water over dough mixture. Mix until all ingredients are combined. Let dough rest for 5 minutes.
6. Form dough into 6 equal rolls (*see note below).
7. (Optional) To a shallow dish, add a small amount of water. To another shallow dish, add sesame seeds. Dip rolls one-by-one in water then sesame seeds to coat the top.
8. Place rolls on a prepared baking dish and bakes for 50 minutes. Turn oven off and crack oven door. Allow rolls to sit inside cooling oven for 10 additional minutes. Remove rolls from oven and allow to fully cool before serving.

Recipe Notes:

I weighed my dough using a food scale. Each roll prior to baking weighed approximately 130-135 grams.

Calories Per Serving: 229

22%Total Fat 14.6g, 8%Total Carbohydrate 23.6g, 81%Dietary Fiber 20.3g

Breakfast Sausage

Prep Time: 5 mins || Cook Time: 10 min

Thanksgiving | Christmas | New Year | Easter

Serves: 12

Cooking Type: Baking

Course: Breakfast

Breakfast Sausage - clean eating is simple with this easy homemade breakfast sausage recipe. Great for freezing too!

Ingredients

- 1 lb ground turkey (or pork or chicken)
- 1 teaspoon Italian seasoning
- 1 teaspoon sage
- 1/2 teaspoon all-purpose salt free blend
- 1/2 teaspoon sea salt
- cooking oil of choice

Instructions

4. Combine ground turkey and seasonings in a bowl. Mix well with your hands and form 12 patties.
5. Heat a large skillet over medium heat. Add cooking oil (avocado, coconut, or olive oil) or ghee to the pan. Add patties to the pan (in batches) and cook 3-4 minutes per side, until nicely browned and cooked through.
6. Remove from pan and drain on paper towels if desired. Serve immediately, refrigerate, or freeze for future use.

Alternative to patties, make ground sausage by cooking ground turkey and spices together in the oil, breaking up into pieces.

Calories: 68kcal | Protein: 7g | Fat: 4g | Saturated Fat: 1g | Cholesterol: 31mg | Sodium: 123mg | Potassium: 80mg | Vitamin A: 30IU | Calcium: 11mg | Iron: 0.5mg

Pizza Breakfast Casserole

Prep Time: 10 Mins // Cook Time: 35 Mins

Thanksgiving | Christmas | New Year | Birthday

Yield: 8

Recipe Type: Breakfast

An easy make-ahead breakfast bake with all the Italian flavors of your favorite pizza!

Ingredients

- 2 tbsp olive oil
- 12 eggs
- 2 tsp Italian seasoning
- 1 tsp sea salt
- 1/2 onion diced
- 1 green pepper diced
- 1 red pepper diced
- 1 lb Ground Italian or Breakfast Sausage if not using turkey sausage, sugar and nitrate free brand
- 10-12 regular or turkey pepperoni, sugar and nitrate free brand
- 1 14.5 can diced tomatoes drained
- Turkey Sausage
- 1 lb lean ground turkey
- 1 tsp fennel seed
- 1 tsp salt
- 2 tsp sage
- 1 tsp thyme
- 1 tsp black pepper
- 1/2 tsp cayenne
- 1/2 tsp garlic powder

Instructions

8. Preheat oven to 350. Spray a 9x13 inch casserole dish with olive oil or avocado oil.
9. Make sausage. Heat a large sauté pan over medium high heat and add 1 tbsp olive oil. If making turkey sausage, add all ingredients and cook 5-7 minutes until no longer pink.
10. If using other sausage, cook 5-7 minutes until browned and cooked through.

11. Add cooked sausage to the bottom of the casserole dish. Using the same pan, add remaining olive oil and chopped onions and peppers.
12. Cook until onion is opaque and beginning to soften, 3-4 minutes. Add onions and peppers to the casserole dish along with the drained canned diced tomatoes.
13. Whisk 12 eggs with the Italian seasoning in a bowl. Pour the eggs over the meat and veggies and stir to combine. Top with pepperonis.
14. Bake for 25-30 minutes until cooked through and the eggs are firm/set. Top with ranch dressing and enjoy! Store in the fridge for up to 5 days.

Veggie Keto Burgers

Prep Time: 15 Mins // Cook Time: 35 Mins

Thanksgiving | Christmas | New Year | Easter

Servings: 6

These are so delicious and super easy to do! I make a huge batch and I freeze them individually in zip lock bags. If you want one or two because they are that GOOD and TASTY you can either toast **them or bake in oven.**

Ingredients:

- Optional: Spaghetti Squash or Sweet potatoes 1 Cup - Optional
- 4 Tbl Psyllium Husk Powder
- 1 Cup Chopped Parsley
- 1 Cup Chopped Cilantro
- 1 Cup chopped Kale
- 2 Cups Green Pea
- 2 Large Yellow or White Onions
- 3 Cups Zucchini
- 1 Cup Sun Dried Tomatoes
- 1/2 Cup Mushrooms
- 1 Cup Peppers
- 10 Cloves Garlic
- 3 Whole Lemons
- 2 Tbl Pink Salt
- 1 Tbl Black pepper
- 2 Tbl Paprika
- 3 Tbl Oregano
- 1 Tbl Dried Dill
- 1 Tbl Mustard
- 1/2 Cup Grape seed Oil or Olive Oil

Instructions:

9. Stir Fry everything together.
10. Add more or less spice as you like.
11. Blend everything together except for the Green Pea.
12. Mix everything well.
13. Form into Shapes
14. Bake on 375F for 12-15 minutes
15. Let cool them pack and store in Freezer.
16. Enjoy!

Low Carb Blueberry Muffins

Prep Time: 10 Mins // Cook Time: 30 Mins

Thanksgiving | Christmas | New Year | Easter

Yield: 12

Serving Size: 1 Muffin

Ingredients

- 1/2 cup coconut flour
- 6 tablespoons psyllium husk
- 1 teaspoon baking powder
- 1/2 teaspoon salt
- 1/2 cup unsweetened sunflower seed butter
- 1/4 cup softened coconut oil, ghee or tallow
- 4 large eggs, room temperature
- 3 tablespoons yacon syrup or 1/3 cup honest syrup
- 1/2 cup non-dairy milk of choice
- 1 teaspoon vanilla extract
- 2 tsp. lemon zest
- 1 cup blueberries

Instructions

9. Preheat oven to 350F. Line a muffin tin with cupcake liners.
10. In a large bowl whisk together the coconut flour, psyllium husk, baking powder and salt.
11. In a separate bowl beat together the sunflower seed butter, coconut oil, eggs, syrup, vanilla and milk until well combined and creamy.
12. Add the wet mix to the dry mix and beat until a dough forms.
13. Add in the blueberries and lemon zest and use a spatula to fold in.
14. Use a ¼ cup scoop per muffin. Bake in the center rack for 25- 30 minutes or until the muffins have risen, round and golden on top.

15. Coconut Flour Blueberry Muffins (paleo, keto, dairy free, nut free)

16. Remove from the oven and let cool. Store in an airtight container at room temperature for up to 5 days.

Recipe Notes:

You can also use Zero Syrup which is vegetable glycerin (a sugar alcohol) and monk fruit or Honest Syrup made of vegetable fiber and monk fruit. While the latter is free of sugar alcohols which is ideal for some, it is high very high in total carbs (fiber). Use 1/4 to 1/3 cup in this recipe instead of Yacon Syrup.

Calories: 176.2, Fat: 12.7g, Carbohydrates: 10.4g, Fiber: 6.5g, Protein: 5.2g

Gluten Free Pumpkin Bread Recipe

Prep Time 15 minutes // Cook Time 50 minutes

Thanksgiving | Christmas | New Year | Easter

Servings 12

Calories 169kcal

A gluten free pumpkin bread recipe made with coconut flour with a taste and texture like the real thing, except it's low carb and completely sugar-free!

Ingredients

- 3/4 cup coconut flour
- 1/2 cup Sukrin Gold packed (or my brown sugar substitute)*
- 3 tbsp whey protein isolate
- 2 1/2 tsp baking powder
- 2 tsp cinnamon
- 1/2 tsp salt
- 6 large eggs
- 4 oz ghee, melted
- 2 tsp vanilla extract
- 1 tsp Stevia Glycerite
- 1 1/2 cup fresh, grated pumpkin (6 oz)

Topping (optional)

- 2 tbsp chopped pecans
- 2 tbsp Sukrin Gold

Instructions

9. Preheat the oven to 350 degrees F and place rack into the middle of the oven. Spray an 8x4 inch loaf pan with baking spray and cut a piece of parchment to fit inside and hand over the sides of the pan (see picture).
10. Pumpkin bread made with coconut flour in a pan with pumpkins and blue napkin.
11. Thoroughly mix the dry ingredients in a medium bowl.
12. Add the wet ingredients and grated pumpkin.
13. Blend with a hand mixer until fully incorporated and spoon into the prepared baking pan. Lift the pan a few inches above the counter and let it fall, knocking out any big air bubbles. Do this 2-3 times.
14. Sprinkle chopped pecans over the top of the bread and gently press into the batter. Sprinkle with the brown sugar substitute.

15. Bake for 50-60 minutes or until a toothpick inserted in the middle comes out clean, but the bread still sounds moist. Let cool in the pan for 5 minutes. Loosen the bread from the ends of the pan and lift the loaf to a cooling rack. Let cool completely.
16. Store in the refrigerator in a plastic bag for up to a week or freeze. Serves 12.

Calories: 169kcal | Carbohydrates: 5g | Protein: 7g | Fat: 13g | Sodium: 227mg | Fiber: 2g

Blackberry Coconut Fat Bombs

Prep Time 5 minutes // Cook Time 5 minutes

Thanksgiving | Christmas | New Year | Easter

Servings 16 small squares

Calories 170kcal

These sugar free blackberry coconut fat bombs are low carb and Paleo. Eat them between meals to stay in ketosis on a ketogenic diet during weight loss.

Ingredients

- 1 cup coconut butter see note for how to make homemade
- 1 cup coconut oil
- 1/2 cup fresh or frozen blackberries can use raspberries or strawberries if desired
- 1/2 teaspoon SweetLeaf stevia drops add a bit more for sweeter taste
- 1/4 teaspoon vanilla powder or 1/2 teaspoon vanilla extract
- 1 tablespoon lemon juice

Instructions

7. Place coconut butter, coconut oil and blackberries (if frozen) in a pot and heat over medium heat just until well combined.
8. In a food processor or small blender, add coconut oil mix and remaining ingredients. Process until smooth. NOTE: Separation may occur if coconut oil mixture is too hot. If using fresh berries, there is no need to cook them with the coconut oil and butter.
9. Spread out into a small pan lined with parchment paper (I used 6x6-inch container)
10. Refrigerate one hour or until mix has hardened.
11. Remove from container and cut into squares.
12. Store covered in the refrigerator.

Notes

- To make coconut butter, place about 2 cups unsweetened dried coconut flakes into food processor and process until butter forms (about 7-8 minutes) 0.8g net carbs
- The amount of berries can be increased for a sweeter and more intense berry taste.

Calories 170 Calories from Fat 168, Total Fat 18.7g 29%|Total Carbohydrates 3g 1%|Dietary Fiber 2.3g 9%|Protein 1.1g 2% |Net Carbs 0.7g| Carbs: 1.6%|Protein: 2.5%

Coconut Lemon Curd Cake

Prep Time: 1 hr 30 mins // Cook Time: 50 mins

Thanksgiving | Christmas | New Year | Easter

Calories: 359 kcal

Servings: 12

A scrumptious and low carb coconut cake filled with a tangy sugar free lemon curd. The lemon curd and cake can be prepared several days in advance and refrigerated. Assemble and frost the cake the day before needed so the lemon curd will have time to set up.

Ingredients

Lemon Curd:

- 1/2 cup fresh lemon juice
- 1/2 cup granular Swerve Sweetener
- 3 large eggs
- 3 large egg yolks
- 3 tbsp. ghee
- 2 tsp arrowroot powder or cornstarch
- Zest from the lemons

Coconut Cake:

- 4 oz unsalted ghee softened
- 4 oz cream cheese softened
- 1/2 cup granular Swerve Sweetener
- 1 tsp coconut extract
- 1/2 tsp vanilla extract
- 1 cup almond flour
- 1 cup coconut flour
- 2 tsp baking powder
- 1/2 tsp salt
- 1/4 tsp xanthan gum
- 4 large eggs cold
- 3 large egg whites cold
- 2/3 cup almond milk cold

Whipped Cream Frosting:

- 1 1/3 cup heavy whipping cream
- 1/3 cup confectioners Swerve Sweetener

- 1/2 tsp vanilla extract
- 1 tsp coconut extract
- 1/8 tsp xanthan gum

Garnish:

- 1/2 cup flaked coconut for the outside of the cake

Raspberries optional

Instructions

Lemon Curd:

5. Mix the Swerve and arrowroot powder together in a small pot.
6. Add the egg yolks and lemon zest, whole eggs, and lemon juice whisking thoroughly between each addition.
7. Turn the heat to medium and whisk until the mixture just begins to thicken. Adjust the heat to medium-low and whisk briskly until the mixture thickens, all at once.
8. Turn off the heat and continue whisking for 1 minute. Whisk in the butter. Strain the mixture into a clean bowl. Cool, cover with cling film and refrigerate overnight or up to 4 days.

Cake:

7. Preheat oven to 350 degrees F and position rack to the lower third. Spray two 6 x 2 -inch round pans (or three 8x1-inch pans) with baking spray and line the bottoms with parchment.
8. Add the first 5 ingredients to a medium bowl and cream until light and fluffy. Add the egg whites and beat again until light and fluffy. In a small bowl, add the remaining dry cake ingredients and whisk to combine and break up any lumps. Add 1/3 of the dry ingredients and beat until incorporated.
9. Add two eggs and beat until light and fluffy. Scrape down the bowl and repeat the procedure ending with the final addition of the dry ingredients. Lastly, add the almond milk and beat, keeping a nice fluffy texture.
10. Divide the batter between the prepared pans and spread with an offset spatula. Lift the pans a few inches off of the counter and drop 2-3 times to knock out any large air bubbles.
11. Place pans in the oven and raise the temperature to 400 degrees F for 10 minutes, then back to 350 degrees for 20-30 minutes more. The cakes are done when firm to the touch but they still sound a little moist. (Cooking time will be less with three 8-inch pans.)

Remove cakes from the oven and cover with a clean tea towel to cool completely.

12. They will sink a bit in the middle. Wrap with cling film and refrigerate until needed.

To Assemble:

5. Whip the heavy whipping cream with the sweetener and flavorings until almost stiff. Sprinkle the xanthan gum over the whipped cream and whip until very stiff and almost clumpy. Put 1/3 of the whipped cream into a pint ziploc bag and snip off 3/8 inch off the corner (or slide a large round open tip into the bag).
6. Remove and reserve 1/4 cup of lemon curd. Mix the remaining lemon curd to loosen it.
7. For 6-inch pans: Slightly slice off the tops to even out the cakes and then slice each cake in half horizontally. Place one cake half on the serving plate and squeeze a ring or dam of whipped cream along the inside edge of the cake. Spread 1/3 of the lemon curd on the cake up to the dam. Top with another layer of cake, pressing lightly to level. Follow the same procedure and repeat. Top with the remaining cake layer.
8. For 8-inch pans: Do the same as above except don't slice the cakes in half. Spread 1/2 of the lemon curd on the bottom cake layer up to the whipped cream dam. Top with another layer of cake and follow the same procedure. Top with the remaining cake layer.

To Decorate:

4. Frost the cake with the whipped cream. Using small handfuls, apply the flaked coconut to the sides of the cake. Stick 4-5 toothpicks into the top and carefully cover the cake in cling film. Refrigerate overnight.
5. Before serving, remove the toothpicks and mix the remaining lemon curd with enough water (2-3 tbsp.) to make a spoonable (but not runny) mixture. Spoon the lemon curd around the top edge of the cake, encouraging it to drip down. Spoon the rest of the lemon curd over the top of the cake and spread gently with the spoon or an offset spatula. Cut and serve.
6. NOTE: This cake is not overly sweet. If you like your desserts sweet, add liquid stevia drops or stevia glycerite to taste. Fresh raspberries make the perfect garnish.

Recipe Notes

Calories: 359, Fat: 32, Carbohydrates: 9, Fiber: 4, Protein: 9, NET CARBS: 4

DESSERT

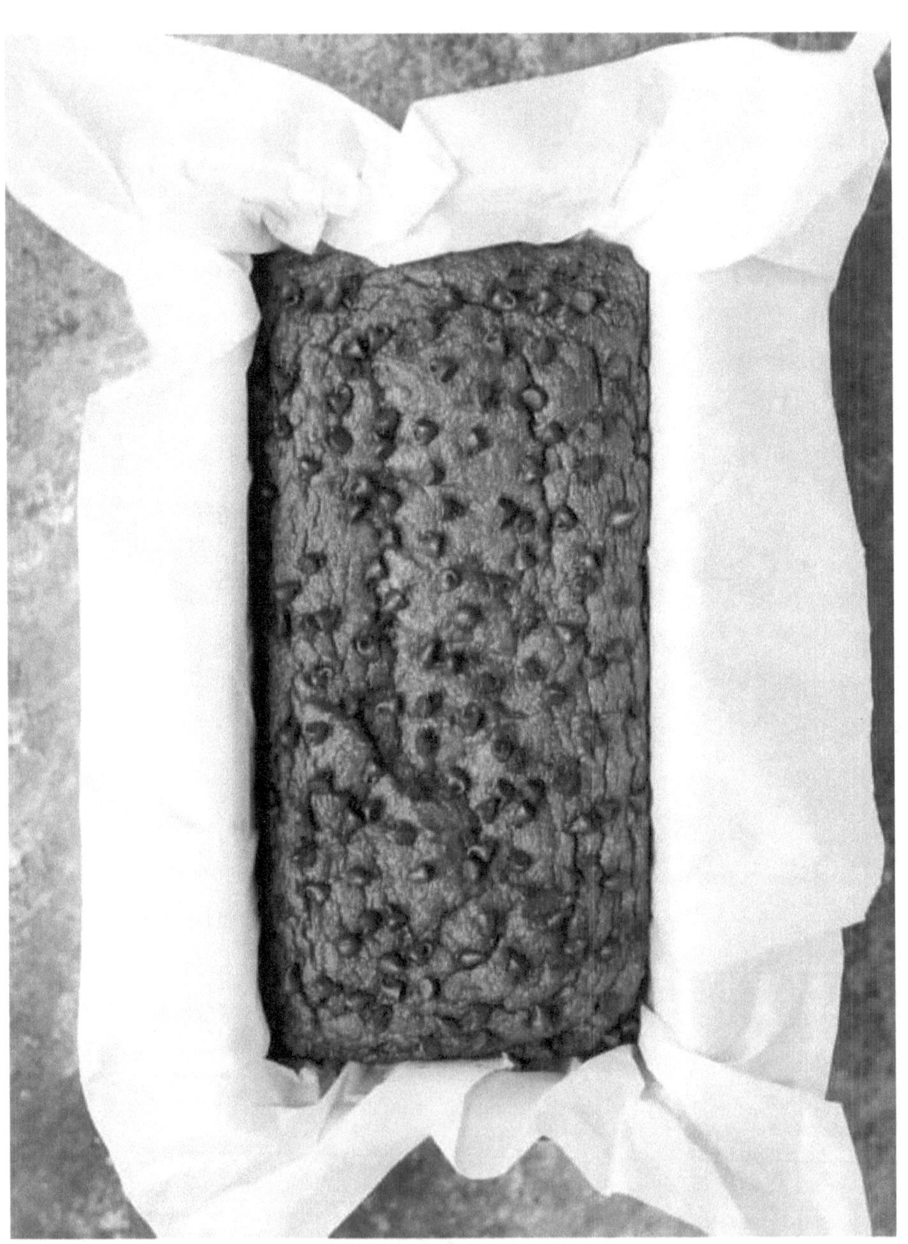

Paleo Pumpkin Bread

Prep time:15 Mins // Cook time: 45 Mins

Thanksgiving | Christmas

yield: 1 (8X4) LOAF

Course: Dessert

Moist and delicious Paleo Pumpkin Bread. Simple, healthy, and low carb pumpkin bread made with almond flour. Easy, gluten free, and filled with fall spices.

Ingredients

- 1 1/2 cups blanched almond flour*
- 1/2 teaspoon kosher salt
- 3/4 teaspoon baking soda
- 2 1/2 teaspoons ground cinnamon
- 1/2 teaspoon ground cloves
- 1/4 teaspoon ground nutmeg
- large eggs
- 3/4 cup Simple Truth Canned Pumpkin — NOT pumpkin pie filling
- 1/4 cup pure maple syrup
- 1 teaspoon pure vanilla extract

Up to 1/2 cup mix-ins: chocolate chips — be sure to use dairy free, Paleo-friendly chocolate chips if necessary, chopped toasted pecans or walnuts, dried cranberries, raisins, chopped dried apricots

Instructions

1. Place a rack in the center of your oven and preheat the oven to 350 degrees F.
2. Lightly coat a 8x4-inch loaf pan with nonstick spray, line with parchment paper so that the paper drapes over the sides like handles, then lightly coat with spray again.
3. In a large bowl, stir together the almond flour, kosher salt, baking soda, cinnamon, cloves, and nutmeg. In a separate bowl, whisk together the eggs, pumpkin, maple syrup, and vanilla.
4. Make a well in the center of the dry ingredients, then pour in the wet. Gently stir, just until combined and the flour disappears. Fold in any desired mix-ins.
5. Scrape into the prepared loaf pan and smooth the top. Bake for 42 to 48 minutes, until a toothpick inserted in the center comes out clean.

6   Place the pan on a wire rack and let cool 30 minutes. Gently lift out the bread with the parchment overhang and place on the rack to finish cooling completely. Slice and enjoy!

Recipe Notes

*Be sure to use blanched almond flour, which is finely ground from blanched almonds that have the skin removed, not coarse almond flour (often called "meal"), which has the brown skins. No other flour can be substituted, as almond flour has very unique properties.

To make your own almond flour:

1   Place blanched, slivered almonds in a food processor and pulse until you have a fine powder.
2   About 1 1/2 cups of slivered almonds will yield the 1 1/2 cups flour needed for the recipe.
3   Be sure to measure before baking. Depending upon your food processor, you may also want to process the almonds in two batches to ensure they blend evenly.

- Store leftovers in an airtight container lined with paper towels in the refrigerator for up to 5 days.
- This bread tastes even better the second day, once the flavors have a chance to marry. Bread can be tightly wrapped and frozen for 3 to 4 months. Let thaw overnight in the refrigerator.

Amount per serving (1 (of 10), without mix-ins) — Calories: 153, Fat: 10g, Saturated Fat: 1g, Cholesterol: 74mg, Sodium: 177mg, Carbohydrates: 11g, Fiber: 2g, Sugar: 6g, Protein: 6g

Sugar-Free Paleo Pecan Snowball Cookies

Prep Time 5 minutes // Cook Time 15 minutes

Thanksgiving | Christmas | New Year | Birthday

Servings 24

Calories 112 kcal

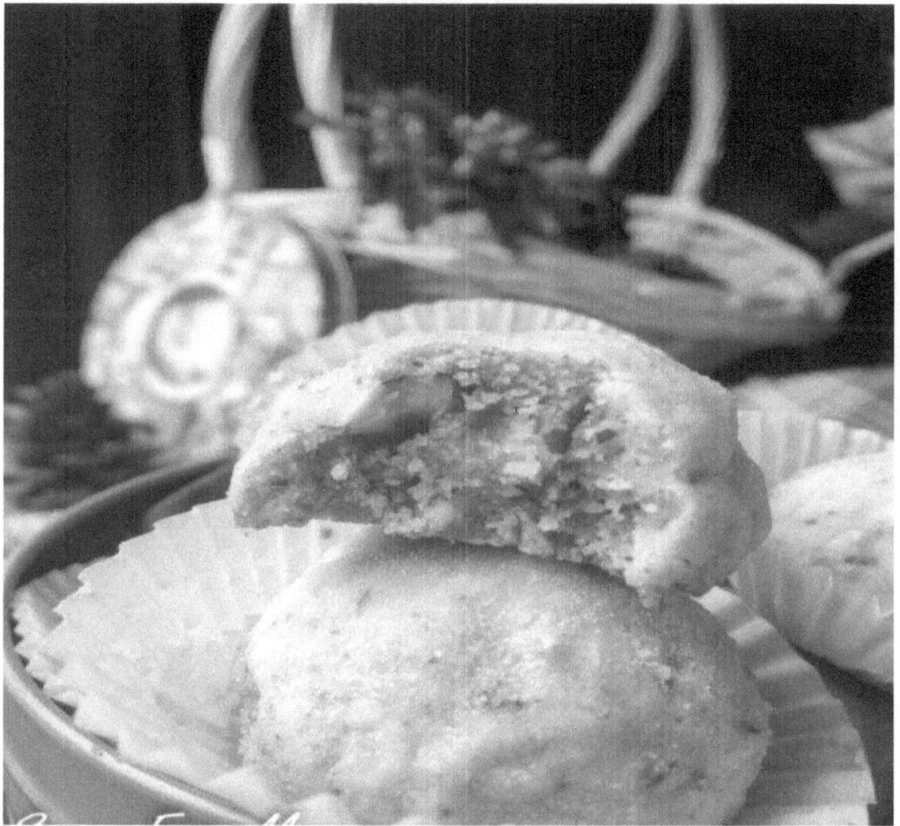

Ingredients

- 3 tbsp Ghee
- 1 1/2 cup almond flour 150 grams
- 1 cup pecans 120 grams, chopped
- 1/2 cup Swerve Confectioners Sweetener 78 grams
- 1 tsp vanilla extract
- 1/2 tsp vanilla liquid stevia
- 1/4 tsp salt

- extra confectioners to roll balls in
- Get IngredientsPowered by Chicory

Instructions

1. Preheat oven to 350 degrees F.
2. Place all ingredients into food processor and process until batter forms a ball. Pulse if needed.
3. Taste batter, adjust sweetener if needed.
4. Line a baking sheet with silpat or parchment.
5. Use a cookie scoop and make 24 mounds.
6. Roll each mound in the palm of your hand.
7. Place in freezer for 20-30 minutes.
8. Place in oven for 15 minutes or until golden around edges.
9. Allow to cool slightly.
10. Once able to handle roll each in some confectioners sweetener.
11. Allow to cool completely before storing in an air tight container.

Recipe Notes

Net Carbs: 1g

Amount Per Serving (1 cookie)

Calories 112Calories from Fat 99Fat 11g17%, Saturated Fat 3g19%, Cholesterol 12mg4%, Sodium 24mg1%, Potassium 16mg0%, Carbohydrates 2g1%, Fiber 1g4%, Protein 1g2%, Vitamin C 0.1mg0%, Calcium 18mg2%.Iron 0.4mg2%

Homemade Coconut Cream Pie Larabars

Prep Time: 5 mins

Thanksgiving | Christmas | New Year | Easter

Servings: 16 small bars

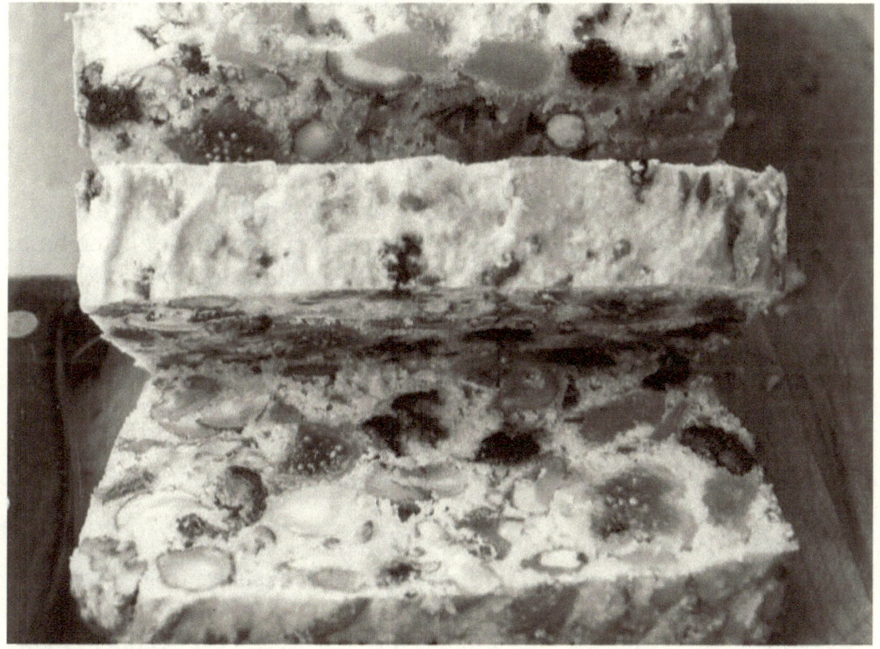

The perfect all natural sweet snack with no added sugar or preservatives.

Author: Tricia

Ingredients

- 2/3 cups raw almonds
- 2/3 cups raw cashews
- 1/2 cup unsweetened shredded coconut
- 1 1/2 tablespoons Coconut Oil
- 12 ounces pitted
- dates, about 1 1/2 cups packed

Instructions

1. Line a loaf pan with parchment paper with enough extra that the paper comes up the sides of the pan. Set aside.
2. In the bowl of a food processor, process the almonds and cashews until finely chopped, leaving a few bigger chunks.
3. Add the coconut, coconut oil, and dates.
4. Process until well blended and holding together.
5. Press the mixture into the prepared loaf pan and use some of the extra parchment paper on the sides to press down on the top of the date bars until smooth.
6. Refrigerate 30 minutes before cutting.
7. Store in the refrigerator for up to several weeks.

Tips for the best paleo fruit and nut bread:

- Remember all the fruits (except the banana) in this bread are dried, fresh won't work in this recipe. Others to try that are not listed here: raisins, peach, prune, mango, strawberries, cherries, papaya.
- Fresh nuts from the shell are far superior to the bagged ones, if you can find them. Raw work best, but if you can only find toasted, that ok, as long as they aren't salted. Other nuts to try that are not listed in the recipe: macadamia, cashew, peanut, and pine nuts.
- I only used flax seeds, but there are so many other great ones out there, like pepitas, chia, sunflower, sesame, etc. Feel free to use what you like.
- I pureed my bananas in my small food processor to get a smooth result. If you choose to hand mash yours, make sure they get really well mashed.
- The bread is delicate, and I found that it worked best to cool it, then wrap it in plastic and refrigerate overnight before slicing. The more finely you chop your fruit and nuts, the easier the bread will be to slice, but I like some chunkiness to the texture. A good sharp serrated bread knife works well.
- If you are toasting, be careful not to over do it, the bread will scorch quickly in a regular toaster. A toaster oven works well too.
- This bread freezes nicely, just be sure to wrap it well.

Healthiest, Super Delicious, Paleo Pumpkin Pie!

Prep Time: 1 mins //Cook Time: 45 mins

Thanksgiving | Christmas | New year| Birthday

Course: Dessert

Servings: 4

Calories: 18 Kcal

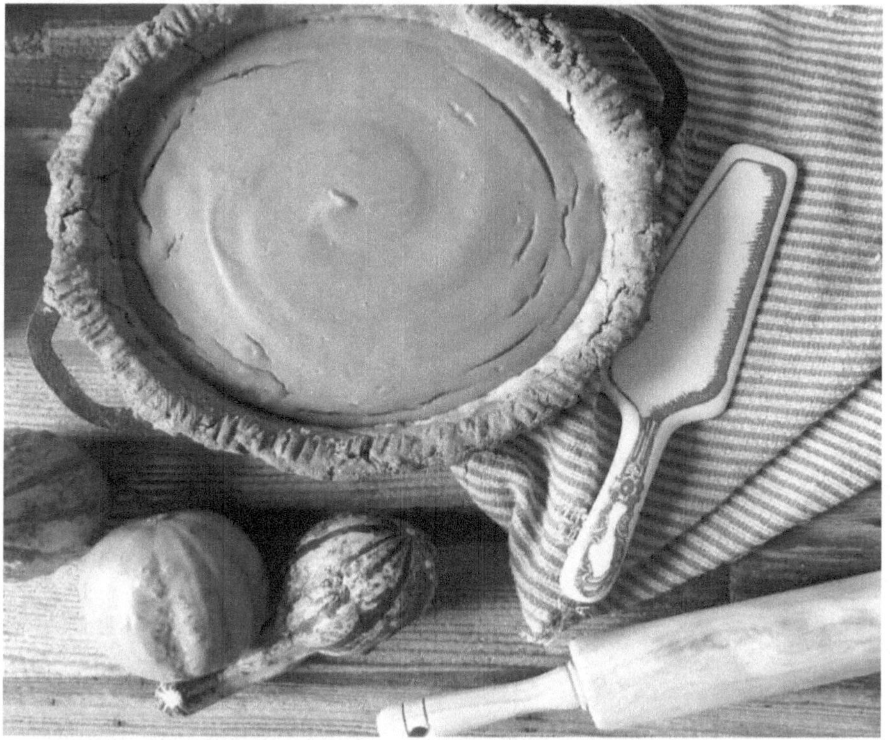

100% PALEO, sweetened only with 5 dates, made with gut healing, clean ingredients, this dessert is sure to win a spot on at any holiday table.

This year Thanksgiving kind of came out of nowhere. We knew we would be jetlagged & unprepared, but I didn't realize how much so.

Ingredients

CRUST

- 1 cup hazelnut meal

- 1/2 cup coconut flour
- 1/2 cup tapioca flour + more for dusting
- 3/4 cup cold lard, cut into 1 inch chunks
- 1 tbsp cold water
- 1 egg
- 1 egg white + water (egg wash)
- pinch salt

FOR FILLING:

- 2 cups roasted Kabocha squash, seeded, no skin
- (I halve, seed and roast it at 400F for 30minutes, let cool and spoon out meat. 1 will do)
- 1 ripe persimmon
- 5 soaked dates, pitted (soak overnight)
- 1/2 cup full fat coconut milk
- 1 tbsp coconut oil
- 1 tbsp Great Lakes Beef gelatin
- 2 eggs
- 1 egg yolk (from the egg wash)
- pinch fine sea salt
- 1/2 tsp cinnamon
- 1/2 tsp ginger
- 1/4 tsp nutmeg
- pinch ground clove
- 1 vanilla bean scrapping

Instructions

For Crust:

1. Sift together flours & salt.
2. Cut lard into flour by pulsing together in food processor until it looks like wet sand.
3. Add in egg and pulse until it forms into a ball.
4. Remove from food processor and wrap in plastic, refrigerate for 30 minutes.
5. Separate two large sheets of parchment paper.
6. Place on counter and dust with tapioca flour.
7. Place the ball in center and pat down into a disk.
8. Dust the disk with tapioca flour and cover with the second sheet.
9. Use a rolling pin to roll out into a 10″ circle.
10. Roll gently in an outward motion.
11. Remove top sheet & carefully place the crust into pie pan.

12. If it cracks, use fingertips to repair the cracks, wet them, it will help.
13. Fold excess over the edge and use a fork to gently imprint on it.
14. Brush with egg wash.
15. In 1/4 inch pattern make holes with a fork in the dough to prevent bubbling.
16. Bake at 400F for 10 minutes. Remove and let cool to the touch.

For filling:

1. In a blender: puree pumpkin, persimmon, dates, coconut milk & oil until smooth.
2. You may need to use prod to keep it moving.
3. Add in spices, salt, vanilla & gelatin, blend in until smooth.
4. Add in egg and blend until smooth.
5. Pour into cooled crust.
6. Bake at 350F for 30 minutes. Let cool to room temperature before serving.
7. Enjoy! I didn't make any, but coconut whipped cream would be pretty sexy on this pie too!

Confetti Turkey Burgers

AIP/ Paleo/Whole /Keto

Prep Time: 20 mins//Cook Time: 35 mins

Thanksgiving | Christmas | New year| Birthday

Yield: 16

Serving Size: 1 Patty

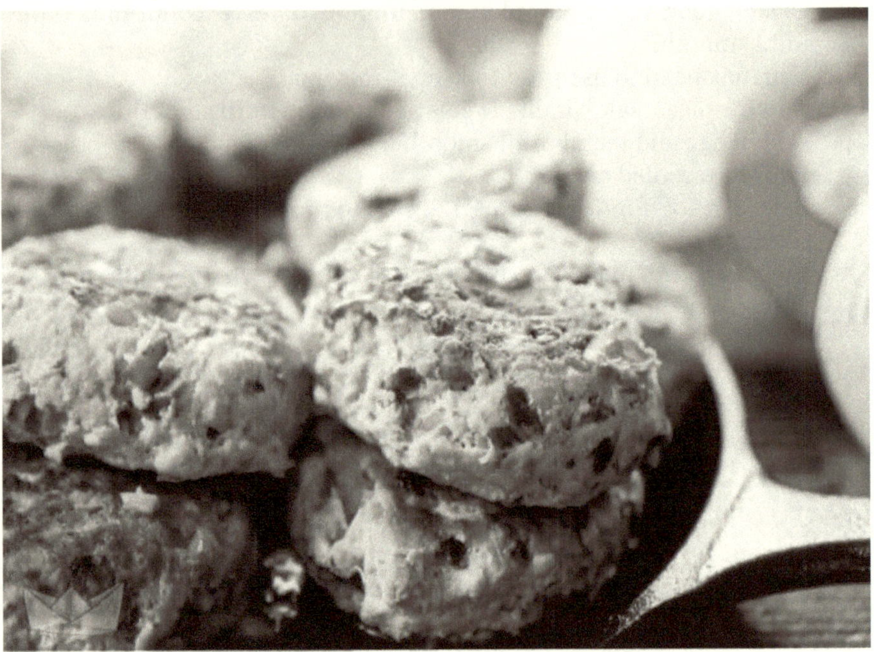

Ingredients

- 4lbs 92%lean ground turkey
- 1 cup minced carrots
- ½ cup finely sliced green onion
- 1 cup minced purple cabbage
- ½ cup minced baby bella mushrooms
- 4 tsp pink Himalayan salt
- 2 tsp ground ginger
- ¼ cup coconut oil (more to cook with)
- 2 rounded tbsp coconut flour

Instructions

1. Heat a large cast iron skillet on medium heat. It will take about 10 minutes to come to temperature.

2. In the meantime, mince and dice and slice all of your veggies. Add them to a bowl with the ground turkey. Add in the oil, ginger and salt.
3. Add in the coconut flour, mix in well then let the mix sit for 5 minutes.
4. Then shape 4 ounces patties and set them on a plate.
5. Lightly oil the skillet. Add 2-3 patties to the skillet at a time. Cook for 5 minutes per side until browned and cooked through. Repeat with all of the patties. Will make around 16 patties.
6. Store in a tupperware or freeze some to have as emergency protein. I like to reheat these stove top as well to get a nice crisp on them. Yum!

Calories: 205, Fat: 12g, Carbohydrates: 4g, Fiber: 1g, Protein: 23g

Lemon Thyme Custard

(Dairy Free, Paleo, Gluten Free)

Prep Time: 10 mins // Cook Time: 15 mins

Thanksgiving | Christmas | New Year | Easter

Yield: 4 1x

Category: dessert

Method: stove top

Serving size: 3 ounces

It's easy to make and something everyone can enjoy. What's extra awesome about this, making it paleo made it a truly nourishing treat. While it's traditional counterpart is made with whole milk and egg yolks, it also calls for a cup of sugar and four tablespoons corn starch. Still gluten free though!

This one is made by whisking together five pastured egg yolks with cashew cream, a quarter cup of maple syrup and half a tablespoon of arrowroot starch Strained with a fine mesh sieve and simmered with lemon peel, cinnamon sticks, and fresh thyme while stirred gently with a wooden spoon. The wooden spoon is a must.

Ingredients

- 2 cups cashew creamer or coconut milk
- 5 egg yolks
- 1/2 tbsp arrowroot starch
- pinch of pink Himalayan Salt
- 1/4 cup maple syrup or 1/3 cup erythritol
- 2 inch piece of lemon rind
- 6 sprigs thyme (small bunch)
- 2 cinnamon sticks
- 1 tsp vanilla extract

Instructions

1. In a large bowl whisk together egg yolks, sweetener, arrowroot starch and a pinch of salt.
2. Add the milk in as you whisk it together, until fully incorporated.
3. Pour the mix through a fine mesh sieve in to a medium sized pot.
4. Add in the lemon rind, thyme and cinnamon sticks. You can tie your thyme together with some string (kitchen safe, to make it easier to remove later).

5. Heat on medium heat, stir with a wooden spoon continuously for about ten minutes.
6. When the mixture begins to coat the back of the wooden spoon, mix in the vanilla extract.
7. Remember to remove the thyme, cinnamon sticks and lemon rind. I used tongs to fish them out.
8. Stir on medium heat for another two to five minutes until thick.
9. Remove from heat.
10. Distribute the custard into ramekins or bowls (about 3, 4 oz a serving).
11. Let them cool. Set in the fridge until serving time.

Recipe Notes:

If you're going to use store bought nut milk, you may have to compensate and add more egg yolks or starch.

Aunt Jen's Pumpkin Bread/Muffins

Dairy-Free, Gluten-Free, Soy-Free

Prep Time 10 minutes// Cook Time 15 minutes

Thanksgiving | Christmas | New Year | Easter

Makes: 6

Ingredients

- 1 1/2 cups White Sugar
- 1 3/4 cups Flour (I used Gluten Free King Arthur 1:1 flour)
- 1 tsp. Baking Soda
- 1/4 tsp. Salt
- 1/2 tsp. Cinnamon
- 1/4 tsp. Nutmeg
- 1/2 cup Oil (I used Canola)
- 2 Eggs
- 1/3 cup Water
- 1 cup 100% Pure Pumpkin (I used canned)

Nuts Optional - Mixed In or Just on Top

Instructions

1. Preheat oven to 350 degrees. Add all of the dry ingredients into a large bowl. Whisk together to ensure they are mixed up.
2. Add the liquids, mix with hand mixer until combined.
3. Pour into greased pans (I sprayed with Avocado Oil) mini loaf pans, large muffin pans, cupcake tins, etc. Bake until done. The toothpick should come out clean.

Christmas Coconut Cookies

Dairy-Free, Gluten-Free, Sugar-Free, Soy-Free, Nut-Free

Prep Time: 15 Mins // Cook Time: 35 Mins

Thanksgiving | Christmas | New Year | Easter

I love those!! You can decorate as you desire - Filled with healthy and Nutritious Ingredients, Real easy to make and I'm sure you have the ingredients already in your kitchen cabinet!

Ingredients:

- 3 Cups Coconut Shreds
- 1 Cup Melted Coconut Oil
- 3 Drops Mint Extract (or any other Extracts as you wish)
- 1/4 Cup Lakanto , Zero Free Maple Syrup (Keto Approved)

Instructions:

1. Melt the coconut oil
2. Mix all the ingredients together with your hands
3. Refrigerate for 30 minutes before shaping
4. start shaping
5. Add any decorations you like to make them more interesting like: Edible Glister, melted chocolate or Caramel (Recipe for my homemade caramel is under "Notes"
6. Store in a sealed container and put in fridge

Paleo Coconut Cupcakes

Dairy-Free, Gluten-Free, Grain-Free, Paleo

Thanksgiving | Christmas | New Year | Easter

Prep Time: 10 Mins // Cook Time: 20 Mins

Servings: 2

Yield: 8 cupcakes

Ingredients

Coconut Cupcakes:

- 1 1/2 cups (120 grams) unsweetened desiccated coconut
- 45 grams (~about 1/2 cup but weigh it!) blanched almond flour
- 2 teaspoons (6 grams) coconut flour
- 3/4 teaspoon baking powder1
- 1/4 teaspoon salt
- 3 large eggs, room temperature
- 1/3 cup (106 grams) honey
- 1/3 cup (80ml) canned, full-fat shaken coconut milk
- 3 tablespoons (42 grams) coconut oil, melted
- 1 1/2 teaspoons coconut or vanilla extract
- Coconut Whipped Cream:
- 1 13.5 ounce (400ml) can of full-fat coconut milk
- coconut sugar or honey, optional

Garnish:

- 1/3 cup toasted coconut
- Easter egg candies, optional (omit for paleo)

Instructions

1. Preheat the oven to 350°F (175°C). Line 8 muffin cups with liners.
2. In a large bowl, mix together the dry ingredients and set aside.

3. In a medium bowl, mix together the wet ingredients (eggs through extract) and combine this with the dry ingredients. Mix just until combined!

4. Fill the cupcake liners so that they're almost full and bake for 20 minutes or until a toothpick inserted in the middle comes out clean.

5. Remove from the oven, let the cupcakes cool for 2 minutes in the tins, and then turn the cupcakes out onto a wire rack to cool completely before frosting.

6. For the coconut whipped cream, put a can of coconut milk in the refrigerator, being careful not to shake it. Let it sit overnight. Take the can out of the refrigerator and scoop out the hardened coconut cream and transfer into a medium mixing bowl. Save the water to drink or to add to a smoothie.

7. Beat the coconut cream using a hand mixer at medium speed until it's the consistency of regular whipped cream. Add coconut sugar or honey, to taste, if desired, and beat on low until well combined.

8. Spread on the cupcakes and add toasted coconut (I just toasted it about 5 minutes after I took out the cupcakes). Add the Easter candies right before serving.

Notes

Make sure to use Grain-Free baking powder, if necessary.

Healthy Banana Pumpkin Cookies (AIP, Paleo, Vegan, Sugar Free)

Prep Time: 15 mins //Cook Time: 10 mins

Thanksgiving | Christmas | New Year | Easter

Course: Dessert, Snacks

Servings: 12 cookies

Calories: 44 kcal

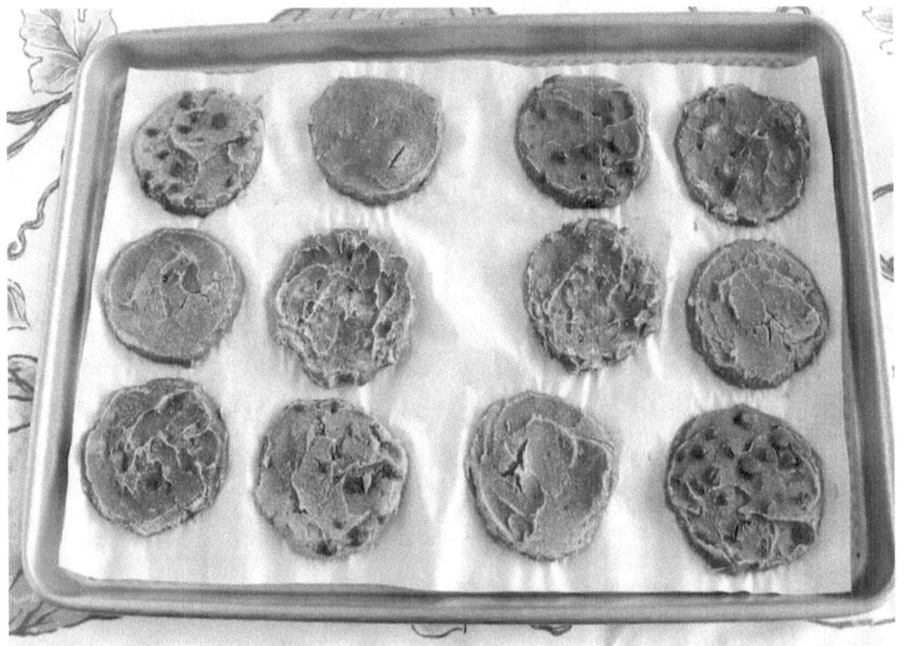

Healthy banana pumpkin cookies are the best fall recipe! This AIP, paleo, vegan and no sugar added recipe makes soft and chewy cookies with a sweet spiced flavor.

Ingredients

- 1 medium banana pureed
- 3/4 cup pumpkin puree
- 1/2 cup tapioca flour
- tbsp coconut flour

- 1/4 tsp baking soda
- 5-7 chopped pitted dates
- 1 tsp pumpkin pie spice or cinnamon (AIP)

Instructions

1. Pre-heat the oven to 350°. Use a blender, food processor or stick blender to mix all ingredients except the dates (or chocolate chips).
2. If using the dates, chop the dates. Add the dates to the batter and stir gently with a spoon. If using chocolate chips, add them to the dough and fold into the dough.
3. Place parchment paper or a silpat on a cookie sheet (you need parchment paper or else the cookies may stick).
4. Place spoonfuls of the cookie dough onto the cookie sheet. The batter will be more moist than regular cookie dough. Use the spoon to shape the batter into a flat circle cookie shape. Repeat until all of the batter is out.
5. Bake the cookies at 350° for about 10 minutes or until a toothpick inserted comes out clean.

Recipe Notes

1. If you are on AIP, you'll want to use chopped dates with this recipe-- it really makes the recipe!
2. If you are not on AIP, you can use chocolate chips in place of dates. I have tried both ways. Usually I'm a chocolate fiend, but I actually prefer dates for this recipe...it really pairs well with the other flavors.
3. If you are on AIP, do not use pumpkin pie spice. Substitute equal amounts cinnamon.
4. I've updated this recipe so you can make it without coconut butter since not everyone has that on hand. However, if you have coconut butter, I would recommend adding 1 tbsp to your cookie dough mixture to further add to the perfect texture.

5   The banana is an important part of this recipe and should not be
    substituted since it adds sweetness and acts as an egg-free binder.
6   Tapioca flour can be substituted with arrowroot or cassava flour.
    The coconut flour cannot be substituted.
7   It's important to use parchment paper or a silpat on the cookie sheet
    when making these so they don't stick.
8   Store these cookies in the refrigerator or freezer. They will last about
    a week in the refrigerator.

Calories 44, Sodium 29mg1%, Potassium 85mg2%, Carbohydrates 10g3%, Fiber 1g4%, Sugar 3g3%, Vitamin A 2390IU48%, Vitamin C 1.5mg2%, Calcium 6mg1%, Iron 0.4mg2%

Salted Caramel Apple Parfaits

Prep Time: 20 minutes // Cook Time: 25 minutes

Thanksgiving | Christmas | New Year | Easter

Yield: 6 parfaits

Category: dessert

Ready for a warm and comforting fall treat? These Autoimmune Paleo (AIP) friendly Caramel Apple Parfaits are just what you're looking for. These parfaits are nut free, gluten free, and dairy free, and full of fall flavor. Store in a mason jar for a pre-portioned, easy to store treat.

Ingredients

Apple Filling

- 2 cups apples, peeled and sliced (you can also use pears or a combo)
- 2 tsp ground cinnamon
- 1 Tbsp coconut oil
- Salted Caramel Sauce
- 1/2 cup pure maple syrup
- 1/2 cup full fat coconut milk, room temperature (be sure your can of coconut milk is well combined, otherwise you may end up with too much cream or too much water)
- 1/2 Tbsp coconut oil
- 1/2 tsp sea salt
- 1/2 tsp vanilla extract (optional)

Coconut Crumble

- 1 batch of my Pumpkin Spice Granola or:
- 2 cups shredded, unsweetened coconut
- 2 Tbsp pure maple syrup
- 2 tsp ground cinnamon
- 1/4 tsp sea salt

Assembly

- 1 batch Apple Filling
- 1 batch Salted Caramel Saunce
- 1 batch Coconut Crumble
- 1 batch Coconut Milk Whipped Cream (this can be purchased from a store or you can make your own using this recipe)

Instructions

Apple Filling

1. Peel and slice your apples and/or pears.
2. Melt coconut oil in a saute pan and add sliced fruit and cinnamon. Stir occasionally until the fruit is soft (about 5-10 minutes).

Salted Caramel Sauce

1. Heat maple syrup over medium low heat for about 5 minutes, stirring constantly. Timing should start with the syrup is bubbling.
2. Be sure to stir constantly, and don't overheat or it will burn.
3. Remove from heat and add remaining ingredients. Stir to combine.
4. Add pan back to heat for about 10 minutes, stirring constantly. The timer should start when the mixture starts to bubble again.
5. Don't bring to a boil, or it will over harden. The mixture should thicken, but won't solidify. Set aside in a jar to cool.

Coconut Crumble

1. Preheat oven to 300 degrees. Line a cookie sheet with parchment paper.
2. Combine ingredients in a bowl until the coconut is well covered with syrup and cinnamon.
3. Spread the mixture evenly across cookie sheet, and bake until it turns golden brown. The coconut will crisp as it cools.

Assembly

1. Drizzle Salted Caramel Sauce around the top of six small glasses. Allow caramel to drizzle down the sides of each glass.
2. Alternate layering Coconut Crumble and Apple Filling in the jars, stopping about 1" from the top.
3. Top each parfait with a small scoop of Coconut Milk Whipped Cream and sprinkle with ground cinnamon.

Savory Breakfast Cookies (flattened biscuits)

Prep time: 15 minutes // Cook time: 40-45 minutes

Thanksgiving | Christmas | New Year | Easter

Yield: 12

Ingredients

- 1/2 cup coconut flour
- 1/2 tsp baking soda
- 1/2 tsp unrefined salt
- 1 tsp dried rosemary
- 1 tsp dried granulated garlic
- 4 Tbsp extra-virgin olive oil
- 6 Tbsp coconut oil
- 4 Tbsp gelatin (Great Lakes brand is from grass-fed cows
- 1 cup room temperature filtered water
- 1/2 Tbsp raw apple cider vinegar
- parchment paper

Instructions

1. Preheat oven to 350F.
2. Prepare your gelatin for use. First, you will have to "bloom" it, then you will melt it. Add water to a small pot and sprinkle/rain gelatin on top, about 1/2 Tbsp at a time in a single layer. Do NOT let it clump or pour it all in one place. You want to spread it out evenly.
3. If not, clumps may form that are difficult to dissolve and the texture in the final product will be negatively affected. Be patient with this part! I use a whisk and vigorously stir the gelatin after each 1/2 Tbsp has been added and wetted.
4. Once all gelatin has been wetted, heat over medium low for several minutes until all gelatin has melted and you have a translucent liquid. Stir occasionally with your whisk until dissolved.
5. While you are waiting on the gelatin to melt, mix all dry ingredients together in a large bowl. I recommend sifting the coconut flour to remove any clumps. Be sure to evenly distribute the baking soda throughout.
6. Once gelatin is completely dissolved, add remaining wet ingredients to gelatin (oils and apple cider vinegar), then pour all wet ingredients into the bowl with your dry ingredients and stir with a large spoon.

7   At first, the batter will seem like it is going to be too runny, but as you stir it the batter will thicken up and soon look like a normal batter.

8   Use your spoon to divide batter into 12 cookies/biscuits onto a parchment paper-lined baking sheet (trust me -- do NOT skip the parchment paper!) Bake at 350F for about 40-45 minutes, or until the cookies are golden and the edges are slightly browned and you can easily lift them with a spatula.

9   If they stick to the paper or come apart in the middle, they are not ready yet. For some reason, the gelatin makes these have a longer cooking time than they would have if made with eggs.

10   Serve immediately and enjoy! Store leftovers in an air-tight container and reheat in the oven for several minutes before serving. I do not recommend eating them cold as they do not have a great texture. They will be crispier the second time they are heated, too.

NOTE: Be sure to wash your pot, whisk, bowl, spoon, and anything else that touched the gelatin right away. If you let it sit, the gelatin will harden and become much harder to clean!

Blueberry Tart (AIP, Paleo, Gluten Free)

Prep Time: 1 hr // Cook Time: 20 mins

Thanksgiving | Christmas | New Year | Easter

Servings: 8 Servings

Course: Dessert

Calories: 305 kcal

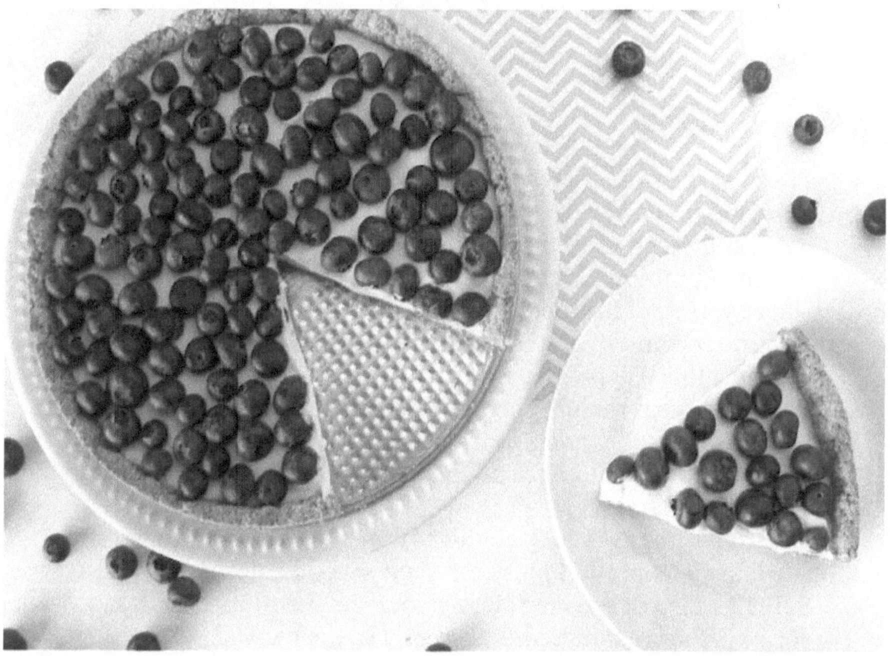

This gluten-free & autoimmune paleo blueberry tart is the perfect
healthy treat! Even if you're not on AIP or the Paleo diet, you'll still
enjoy this fresh and tasty tart!

Ingredients

Crust:

- 1 cup dates pitted
- 3 tbsp coconut oil (+ 1 tbsp for greasing the pan)
- 3/4 cup arrowroot flour
- 1/4 cup coconut flour
- 1/4 tsp baking soda
- 1/4 tsp sea salt

- 1/2 tsp vanilla extract
- 3 tbsp unsweetened applesauce

Filling:

- 1 14 oz. can coconut cream (or 1 13.5 oz. can full-fat coconut milk refrigerated overnight)
- 1 tsp vanilla extract
- Dash sea salt
- 1 tbsp maple syrup (optional)
- 11 oz. blueberries (about 1 1/2 cups)

Instructions

To make the crust:

1. Pre-heat the oven to 350°F.
2. In a food processor or high powered blender (like a vitamix) add the dates and blend until they are finely chopped almost into a paste (about 1-2 minutes). The pureed dates may stick into a ball--this is where you want to stop.
3. Add the coconut oil to the food processor and blend for about 30 seconds, this will break up the dates.
4. Then add the remaining crust ingredients (arrowroot, coconut flour, baking soda, salt, vanilla extract and apple sauce) to the food processor and blend until all the ingredients are fully mixed (about 1-2 minutes).
5. Stop and scrape down the sides of the food processor to get any stuck ingredients and pulse for a few seconds more.
6. Spread 1 tbsp of coconut oil to grease the 8 or 9 Inch Tart pan. Then sprinkle the crust ingredients evenly in the pan.
7. Use your hands to press the crust dough evenly into the pan mold, taking care to press the dough all the way to the tops of the sides.
8. Once the dough is firmly and evenly pressed into the tart pan, place it into the oven for 15-20 minutes or until the sides have started to get golden brown.
9. Then remove the crust from the oven and allow to cool for about 30 minutes or until it is cool to the touch.

Filling:

1. To make the filling you'll need either 1 14 oz. can of unsweetened coconut cream or 1 13.5 oz. can full-fat coconut milk refrigerated overnight.
2. You'll need to use a can of full-fat coconut milk--light coconut milk or boxed coconut milk will not work.

3 If you're using the coconut cream, you can scoop the whole thing out of the can into a bowl. For refrigerated coconut milk, you can scoop the coconut cream out of the top into a bowl and leave the clear liquid at the bottom (you can discard the liquid or use it in smoothies).

4 The coconut cream will be hard. Use a whisk to break it up and gently whip it until it becomes the consistency of whipped cream. Add the vanilla and a dash of salt to the coconut cream and mix it.

5 You can also add maple syrup to the coconut cream to make it sweeter if you prefer--I didn't add any sweetener to the coconut cream and for me the crust and blueberries were sweet enough.

6 Once the crust has cooled, scoop the coconut cream into the crust. Then put the crust and coconut cream in the refrigerator to let the coconut cream set (about 10-20 minutes).

7 If you touch the coconut cream with your finger and it makes a small dent that stays in place, then it is set. Remove the crust from the refrigerator.

8 Add the blueberries evenly over the coconut cream and you're all set! The tart is ready to be eaten. Keep any leftovers in the refrigerator since the coconut cream can soften.

Calories 305Calories from Fat 162

Fat 18g28%, Saturated Fat 15g94%, Sodium 122mg5%, Potassium 271mg8%, Carbohydrates 36g12%, Fiber 4g17%, Sugar 17g19%, Protein 2g4%, Vitamin A 20IU0%, Vitamin C 4.8mg6%, Calcium 21mg2%, Iron 1.2mg7%

No-Churn, Two Ingredient Pumpkin Ice Cream

Thanksgiving | Christmas

Serves: Makes 4 servings (or 2 ice-cream-lover sized servings)

Ingredients

- 4 large or 6 small very ripe bananas (lots of black spots), frozen
- ½ cup fresh or canned pumpkin puree (this canned pumpkin doesn't have undisclosed ingredients like many supermarket canned pumpkin!)

Optional: raw honey, pure maple syrup, non-irradiated cinnamon or chocolate chips (I love these chocolate chips, they are dairy and soy free!)

Instructions

1. Blend the frozen bananas and pumpkin together in a high speed blender or food processor until creamy.
2. The bananas must be pre-frozen even if you are going to freeze the ice cream after blending.
3. Taste and add some sweetener, like maple syrup, if desired. Cinnamon and chocolate chips can also be blended in, yum!
4. Serve immediately for soft serve texture or freeze for at least 4 hours for a firmer ice cream.
5. If ice cream is in the freezer for a while, let it soften for about 5 minutes at room temperature before serving.

Pumpkin Spice Paleo Pancakes

Prep Time: 5 mins //Cook Time: 15 mins

Thanksgiving | Christmas | New year| Birthday

Course: Dessert

Servings: 3

Calories: 18 Kcal

Ingredients

- 1/4 cup nut milk (I used cashew milk)
- 2 large eggs
- 1/2 tsp Honey (or preferred liquid sweetener)
- 1 tsp vanilla extract
- 1 tsp apple cider vinegar
- 1/2 cup fine ground blanched almond meal
- 3 level tbsp Otto's Cassava Flour
- 1/4 tsp salt
- 1 tsp baking soda

Pumpkin Spice Seasoning (optional, leave out for plain pancakes)

- 1/2 tsp cinnamon
- 1/2 tsp ground ginger
- 1/4 tsp nutmeg

OTHER

- Tin Star Brown Ghee for cooking
- 1/4 cup chopped pecans (optional)

For topping

- Extra pecans
- 1 tsp Tin Star Brown Ghee
- 1/2 tsp Honey Drizzle on top (Or maple syrup)

Instructions

1. You will need two bowls, a spatula and a griddle or skillet.
2. In one bowl, add all the wet ingredients (eggs, milk, honey, vanilla, vinegar). Whisk to combine. Don't over mix.
3. In another bowl whisk together the dry ingredients, except the pecans.

4. Add the dry ingredients to the wet and mix with a spatula to combine.
5. Fold in the chopped pecans, if you're using them.
6. Heat the skillet or griddle on medium-high heat.
7. Drop a little ghee down, use a 1/4 cup scoop to drop the pancake batter.
8. Will make 4 medium pancakes.
9. Pour batter, once the edges are cooked and there are little bubbles, gently flip the pancake. Cook for another 1-3 minutes.
10. I usually cook my pancakes in a 6″ skillet, one at a time so I don't mess them up.
11. Stack, top with extra ghee, pecans and or honey or maple.
12. Enjoy!

Recipe Notes:

If you need eight pancakes, I would make two batches instead of doubling the batter if you want 8 pancakes because the cassava flour does not duplicate well in recipes.

Pumpkin Cheesecake Bars

Prep Time: 15 minutes // Cook Time: 40 minutes

Thanksgiving | Christmas | New Year | Easter | Halloween

Course: Dessert

Serves: 12 bars

We picked up a few cans of pumpkin puree and set out to create a few holiday recipes our readers are sure to love. First up, a simple recipe for low carb & sugar-free Pumpkin Cheesecake Bars with cream cheese frosting that'll blow your friends and family away. They're appropriate for school bake sales, Halloween, an after-dinner family treat or as a Thanksgiving dessert.

Ingredients

Crust

- 2 cups whole pecans
- 1 tsp cinnamon
- 1 tbsp coconut oil
- 10-15 drops liquid stevia
- 1 pinch sea salt

Filling

- 8 oz. cream cheese
- 1/4 cup heavy cream
- 10 oz. pumpkin puree
- 2 tsp vanilla extract
- 20 drops liquid stevia
- 1/2 cup So Nourished powdered erythritol sweetener
- 1/4 tsp pumpkin pie spice
- 1 tsp cinnamon
- 1 pinch salt
- 2 large eggs

Frosting

- 2 oz. cream cheese
- 2 tbsp heavy cream
- 1/4 cup powdered erythritol sweetener
- 1/2 tsp vanilla extract

Instructions

1. Preheat the oven to 350°F. Combine all the crust ingredients in a food processor and pulse until the pecans are a fine crumb texture. Don't over process or you'll end up with pecan butter!
2. Line a 9x6-inch baking dish with parchment paper, letting two sides spill over for easy removal. Press the crust into the dish, making one even layer. Bake for 12 minutes, then let cool.
3. Meanwhile, using an electric hand mixer, beat the cream cheese and heavy cream until fully combined and even throughout. Then, add in the pumpkin puree, vanilla extract and liquid stevia and combine.
4. Add in the erythritol, pumpkin pie spice, cinnamon and a pinch of salt and combine.
5. Next, add in one egg at a time, incorporating each before adding another.
6. Once the crust has cooled a bit, pour the pumpkin cheesecake batter into the baking dish. Reduce the heat in the oven to 325°F and bake for 25-30 minutes. The middle of the pumpkin cheesecake should be a bit wobbly after baking. Refrigerate for 6 hours or, ideally, overnight.
7. To make the frosting, combine all the frosting ingredients and beat with an electric hand mixer until light and fluffy.
8. Frost the top of the cheesecake bars or add a dollop to each one after slicing. Enjoy!

273 Calories, 25g of Fat, 4g of Protein, 4.5g of Net Carbs

Low Carb Keto Pumpkin Cheesecake

Prep Time 15 minutes // Cook Time 55 minutes

Thanksgiving | Christmas | New Year | Easter

Course: Dessert

Calories 280 kcal

Servings 16 slices

Serving size: 1 slice (1/16 of recipe)

An unbelievably smooth, decant keto pumpkin cheesecake! This easy low carb pumpkin cheesecake recipe just might become your favorite low carb pumpkin dessert ever.

Ingredients

Almond Flour Cheesecake Crust

- 1 1/2 cup coconut flour
- 1/2 cup Vital Proteins Collagen Peptides (or whey protein powder)
- 3 tbsp Erythritol
- 1/3 cup coconut oil
- 1 tsp Vanilla extract

Pumpkin Cheesecake Filling

- 24 oz Paleo Cream cheese (softened)
- 1 cup Pumpkin puree
- 1 1/4 cup Powdered erythritol
- 3 large Eggs (at room temperature)
- 1 tsp Pumpkin pie spice
- 1/2 tsp Cinnamon
- 1 tsp Vanilla extract

Instructions

1. Preheat the oven to 350 degrees F (177 degrees C). Line the bottom of a 9 in (23 cm) springform pan with parchment paper. (You can also try greasing well.)
2. To make the almond flour cheesecake crust, stir the almond flour, collagen or protein powder, and erythritol together.

3. Whisk together the melted oil and vanilla, then stir into the dry ingredients, pressing with the spoon or spatula, until well combined. The dough will be slightly crumbly.
4. Press the dough into the bottom of the prepared pan. Prick gently with a fork all over. Bake for about 12-15 minutes, until barely golden. Let cool at least 10 minutes.
5. Meanwhile, beat the cream cheese and powdered sweetener together at low to medium speed until fluffy. Beat in the pumpkin puree, pumpkin pie spice, cinnamon and vanilla. Beat in the eggs, one at a time. (Keep the mixer at low to medium the whole time; too high speed will introduce too many air bubbles, which we don't want.)
6. Pour the filling into the pan over the crust. Smooth the top with a spatula. (Use a pastry spatula for a smoother top if you have one that fits into the pan.)
7. Bake for about 40-50 minutes, until the center is almost set, but still jiggly.
8. Remove the cheesecake from the oven. If the edges are stuck to the pan, run a knife around the edge. (But, do not remove the springform edge just yet.)
9. Cool the cheesecake in the pan on the counter to room temperature, then refrigerate for at least 4 hours (preferably overnight), until completely set. (Do not try to remove the cake from the pan before chilling.)

Serve with whipped cream and/or a sprinkle of cinnamon.

Calories280, Fat24g, Protein10g, Total Carbs6g, Net Carbs5g, Fiber1g, Sugar2g

Low Carb Spiced Pumpkin Muffins

Prep Time: 10 mins // Cook Time: 25 mins

Thanksgiving | Christmas | New Year | Easter | Halloween

Yield: 12

Serving Size: 1

Category: desserts

Method: baking

Dairy and nut free

Ingredients

PUMPKIN MUFFIN

- 1 heaping cup pumpkin puree (100% pumpkin, unsweetened)
- ¼ cup ghee or coconut oil
- 2 teaspoons Ceylon cinnamon
- 2 teaspoons garam masala
- 1 teaspoon baking soda (or aluminum and corn free baking powder)
- ½ teaspoon pink Himalayan salt
- 1 teaspoon vanilla extract
- 5 large eggs
- 1/3 cup rounded granulated sweetener or 30 drops liquid stevia/ 2 tsp stevia glycerite
- 1/3 cup coconut flour
- 1/3 cup rounded ground flax seed
- (golden flax will produce lighter muffins, regular flax meal will produce darker muffins like photographed)

TAHINI SWIRL

- 2 heaping tablespoons tahini
- 1 tablespoon toasted sesame oil
- 1 teaspoon granulated sweetener
- Pinch of salt

Instructions

1. Pre-heat the oven to 350F.
2. Add cupcake liners to the muffin tin and lightly spray with coconut oil or another nonstick cooking spray.
3. Combine all of the pumpkin muffin ingredients in a large bowl and insert an immersion blender or hand mixer.

4. Blend up to combine until thick batter forms.
5. Use a ¼ measuring cup or scoop to distribute the batter to each muffin mold.
6. In a small bowl mix together the tahini swirl ingredients until smooth. Add a teaspoon to each muffin and use a toothpick to swirl it around.
7. Bake the muffins for 25-28 minutes. Remove from the oven, and let cool to room temperature on a rack before handling.

Calories: 135, Fat: 11g, Carbohydrates: 7g, Fiber: 4g, Protein: 4g

Low Carb Chocolate Cranberry Bundt Cake with Sherry Cooking Wine

Prep Time: 40 minutes // Cook Time: 45 minutes

Thanksgiving | Christmas | New Year | Easter | Halloween

Yield: 8 slices.

Category: Dessert

Method: Bake

Cuisine: American

Are you looking for the perfect keto holiday dessert? This low carb chocolate cranberry bundt cake with sherry cooking wine is the perfect low carb holiday dessert recipe and it is nut free!

Ingredients

- ¾ cup + 1 tsp (86g) coconut flour, divided
- ½ cup (4 oz) coconut oil
- ¼ cup + 3 tbsp (35g) unsweetened cocoa powder
- ¾ cup (144g) classic monk fruit sweetener
- 2 tsp cream of tartar
- 1 tsp baking soda
- ½ tsp (1g) espresso powder
- ½ tsp salt
- ¼ tsp xanthan gum
- 6 eggs
- 200g fresh cranberries
- 1 tbsp (15mL) Holland House Sherry Cooking Wine
- ½ tsp pure vanilla extract

Materials:

- 12 cup Bundt pan

Instructions

1. Preheat oven to 350 degrees and spray Bundt pan with nonstick cooking spray and sprinkle 1 tsp coconut flour inside to lightly coat surface of Bundt pan (this step will help to ensure the cake does not stick to the inside of the pan after baking).

2. In a microwave-safe bowl in the microwave, melt oil. Stir cocoa powder into melted oil until well-combined. Set aside.
3. In a large mixing bowl, whisk together remaining ¾ cup (84g) coconut flour, monk fruit sweetener, cream of tartar, baking soda, espresso powder, salt, and xanthan gum. Add eggs, cranberries, cooking wine, and vanilla extract and, using an electric mixer, mix ingredients together until fully incorporated.
4. Pour in melted chocolate and oil mixture and, with an electric mixer set to the highest speed, mix the mixture until dough is thick and fluffy. Transfer dough to the prepared Bundt pan. Knock Bundt on hard surface multiple times to spread the dough into even layer, smoothing the top as necessary with a rubber spatula.
5. Transfer Bundt pan to the middle rack of oven and bake, uncovered, for 30 minutes. After 30 minutes, loosely cover Bundt pan with foil and continue to bake until a toothpick can be poked into the cake and come out cleanly about 15 additional minutes.
6. Remove pan from oven, leaving foil covering intact on the pan, allowing the cake to cool at room temperature for 20 minutes. After, remove foil, cover pan with hard surfaces, such as a cutting board, and carefully flip the pan over to remove the cake from pan.
7. Allow cake to fully cool before serving.

CHECK OUT ALL OF THE DIETS THIS DELICIOUS CRANBERRY BUNDT CAKE IS COMPLIANT WITH!

- Keto and Low Carb: A ketogenic dieter's cake dream come true, this easy cranberry Bundt cake is super low carb, only containing 5.5 grams of net carbs per serving.
- Nut Free: This recipe is free of nuts and nut products, making it safe to consume for those with nut allergies and intolerances.
- Gluten Free: This cake is great for those with gluten sensitivities because it contains no wheat, barley, or rye!
- Grain Free: Free of quinoa, cornmeal, or oats, this recipe is great for those who do not consume grains.
- Primal: This cake adheres to primal diet restrictions.
- Vegetarian: If you adhere to a vegetarian lifestyle, this cake is for you! There are no meat products within this recipe.
- Refined Sugar Free: This recipe contains no refined sugar

Pumpkin Caramel Bundt Cake

Prep Time: 10 mins // Cook Time: 1 hr

Thanksgiving | Christmas | New Year | Easter | Halloween

Course: Dessert

Servings: 1 cake

Calories: 212 kcal

Serves: 16.

Each serving has 5.21g

All the best flavors of fall in this delicious low carb Pumpkin Spice Bundt Cake with a sugar-free caramel glaze. Grain-free and keto friendly.

Ingredients

Cake:

- 2 1/2 cups almond flour
- 1/2 cup coconut flour
- 2/3 cup Swerve sweetener
- 1/3 cup unflavored whey protein powder
- 1 tbsp baking powder
- 2 tsp cinnamon
- 1/2 tsp salt
- 1 tsp ginger
- 1/4 tsp cloves
- 1 1/2 cups pumpkin puree
- 4 large eggs
- 1/4 cup melted coconut oil
- 1/2 to 2/3 cup water
- 1 tsp vanilla extract

Glaze:

- 1/4 cup coconut oil
- 1 tsp molasses for color and flavor
- 1/2 cup powdered Swerve sweetener
- 1/2 tsp caramel flavour
- 2 tbsp whipping cream

Instructions

Cake:

1. Preheat oven to 325F and grease a 9-inch bundt pan very well.
2. In a large bowl, whisk together the almond flour, coconut flour, sweetener, protein powder, baking powder, cinnamon, salt, ginger, and cloves.
3. Stir in pumpkin puree, eggs, oil, 1/2 cup water, and vanilla extract. If your puree is very thin, you probably won't have to add more water.
4. If it is thicker, add enough water to make the batter spreadable (it should not be so thin as to be pourable).
5. Transfer batter to prepared bundt pan and bake 55 to 60 minutes, or until cake is set and a tester inserted in center comes out clean.
6. Remove and let cool 15 minutes, then transfer to a wire rack to cool completely.

Glaze:

1. In a small saucepan over low heat, melt oil with molasses or yacon syrup, stirring until smooth.
2. Remove from heat and stir in powdered sweetener, caramel extract and whipping cream. Drizzle over cooled cake.

Recipe Notes

Food energy: 212kcal, Total fat: 16.47g, Calories from fat: 148, Cholesterol: 65mg, Carbohydrate: 9.19g, Total dietary fiber: 3.98g, Protein: 7.61g, Erythritol: 7.5g

Ice Cream Pre workout

Prep Time: 15 Mins // Cook Time: 15 Mins

Thanksgiving | Christmas | New Year | Easter | Halloween

Servings: 4

Recipe Type: Dessert

Ingredients

- 4 Cans Coconut Cream (Organic)
- 2 Tsp. Vanilla Extract
- 1 Tbl Cinnamon
- 1/2 Cup Coconut Shreds (Optional) - Don't blend that, just stir into Ice cream when blended.
- 2-4 Tbl Sweetener of choice (Stevia, Monk Fruit_ or any other of your choice.
- 4-5 Scoops of the Vanilla
- You can make this into a Chocolate flavor by just adding 5 Tbl of cocoa powder with 1 Tsp. Mint Extract instead of Vanilla Extract

Instructions:

1. Place a large pan in your freezer.
2. In a blender add the full ingredients, blend till nice and smooth.
3. Transfer the Ice cream to the large pan or Loaf pan that was in your freezer, Pour and transfer back into the freezer.
4. You can enjoy this amazing Ice cream after 30 minutes! Please let it thaw for about 5-10 minutes before eating and wet your Ice cream scoop for a smooth round texture!
5. Enjoy!

Keto Key Lime Pie Recipe

Prep Time: 15 Minute // Cook Time: 20 Minutes

Thanksgiving | Christmas

Servings: 6 Slices

Calories: 118 Kcal

Recipe Type: Dessert

Keto Key Lime Pie an easy to prep no bake lime pie recipe that is perfect for when you just cannot turn your oven on in the summertime. Very refreshing, satisfying and made without sugar so you can enjoy it guilt free and is simple to throw together. Perfect for parties when you have to prep many dishes.

Ingredients:

Crust

- 192 g almond flour or meal
- 1/4-1/2 cup powdered xylitol (or sweetener of choice, to taste)
- 1 tsp. cinnamon
- 1/4 tsp. kosher salt
- 56 g melted ghee/coconut oil

Key Lime Filling

- 400 g avocado about 3
- 250 g coconut cream chilled
- 2 tbsp. freshly grated key lime zest
- 80 ml freshly squeezed key lime juice (to taste)
- 1/3-1/2 cup powdered xylitol (or sweetener of choice, to taste)
- 1/4-1/2 tsp. kosher salt to taste

Instructions

Crust

1. Lightly toast almond flour in a skillet or pan over medium heat, until fully golden and fragrant (2-4 minutes). This is very important taste-wise.
2. Transfer toasted almond flour to a medium bowl, and mix in sweetener, cinnamon and salt.

3. Add in oil, mix until thoroughly combined and press into an 8 or 9-inch pie dish.
4. Allow to come to room temperature and freeze while you make the pie filling.

Key Lime Filling

1. Blend all the filling ingredients, starting with the lower amounts, together using an immersion blender (or high speed blender) until creamy smooth.
2. Taste for sweetness, tanginess, seasoning and adjust accordingly. Key limes can vary a lot in taste, so start with the lower amount and add to taste.
3. Spread the key lime filling over the graham crust lined pie and refrigerate preferably overnight the key lime kick becomes so much better.
4. But if in a pickle you can always pop it in the freezer for an hour or so. Keep in the fridge for 3-4 days and frozen for a month or two.
5. If you like, serve the pie topped with a bit of whipped cream and slices of lime for additional garnish.

Amount Per serving (1 slice)

Calories 297, Calories from Fat 252, Total Fat 28 g, Saturated Fat 12 g, Cholesterol 12 mg, Sodium 160 mg, Potassium 284 mg, Total Carbohydrates 8 g, Dietary Fiber 5 g, Sugars 1 g, Protein 5 g

BLENDED ICED COFFEE

Prep Time: 3 mins ||

Thanksgiving | Christmas | Birthday

Serves: 1

Cooking Type: Baking

Course: Dessert

calories: 115 KCAL

Ingredients

- 1/3 cup coffee concentrate chilled
- 1/4 cup coconut milk
- coffee ice cubes about 1 oz each
- 1 scoop collagen

Instructions

MAKING COLD BREW CONCENTRATE

1. Combine 1/2 cup coarsely ground organic coffee with 30 oz of cold water. If you prefer your coffee dark, increase the amount of grounds to 1 cup.
2. Let your coffee sit for 12-18 hours. The longer it sits, the stronger it gets.

MAKING COFFEE ICE CUBES

1. Add your cold brew to an ice cube tray and freeze for 4-5 hours.

HOW TO MAKE BLENDED ICED COFFEE

2. Combine coffee ice cubes, milk, cold brew concentrate, and collagen in a blender.
3. Blend on high for 1-2 minutes or until the coffee is creamy and smooth.

Note

- Each ice cube in the tray I used is 3/4 oz.
- If your blender struggles with actually blending ice, let the coffee cubes sit for 10 minutes with the milk and cold brew. This will soften them up a little bit to make for easier blending, while still giving the coffee an icy base.

- You can use whatever milk works best for your dietary needs. Coconut will be lovely and creamy or use almond milk to make an iced coffee with almond milk.
- Once you've strained your cold brew, get another batch started and make more ice cubes.

Paleo Pumpkin Pie Recipe

Prep Time: 10 mins || Cook Time: 50 min

Thanksgiving | Christmas | Halloween

Serves: 8 slices

Cooking Type: Baking

Course: Dessert

Serving Size: 9 inch

The best paleo pumpkin pie recipe for the holidays! It's easy to make and a real crowd pleaser.

Ingredients

For the crust

- 125 grams almond flour about 1-1/4 cups
- 3 tablespoons organic ghee or coconut oil
- pinch of sea salt

For the pie

- 1 15- ounce can organic pumpkin
- 3/4 cups coconut milk
- 1/2 cup honey
- 3 eggs
- 2 teaspoons pumpkin pie spice
- 1/4 teaspoon salt

Instructions

1 Preheat oven to 325 degrees.
2 Mix crust ingredients until dough forms. Press into pie plate and bake for 10 minutes. Set aside to cool.
3 Add filling ingredients to food processor and process until smooth. Pour the filling into the crust and bake for 50 minutes, or until filling is just set. Cover crust with pie crust shield or foil if it browns too quickly.
4 Cool completely and refrigerate 2 hours.

Calories: 288kcal | Carbohydrates: 26g | Protein: 6g | Fat: 19g | Saturated Fat: 8g | Cholesterol: 75mg | Sodium: 102mg | Potassium: 197mg | Fiber: 3g | Sugar: 19g | Vitamin A: 8915IU | Vitamin C: 2.8mg | Calcium: 65mg | Iron: 2.6mg

One-Bowl Blueberry Muffins

Prep Time: 10 mins || Cook Time: 20 min

Thanksgiving | Christmas | New Year | Easter |

Serves: 12 muffins

Cooking Type: Baking

Course: Dessert

These keto blueberry muffins have a crisp top and a soft, fluffy inside! They have a sweet nutty flavor thanks to almond butter and almond flour, and are loaded with plenty of juicy sweet blueberries. They're paleo, gluten-free, dairy-free, and low carb.

Ingredients

- 3 eggs room temp
- 1/2 cup smooth almond butter (a drippier one is best for this recipe)
- 2 Tbsp dairy-free milk almond or coconut
- 1/2 cup erythritol
- 2 tsp pure vanilla extract
- 1 Tbsp lemon juice
- 1 1/4 cups blanched almond flour
- 3/4 tsp baking soda
- 1/4 tsp sea salt
- 1 cup blueberries divided

Instructions

1. Preheat your oven to 325 and line a 12 cup muffin pan with parchment liners.
2. In a large mixing bowl, whisk together the eggs, almond butter, milk, erythritol, vanilla, and lemon juice.
3. Add in the almond flour, baking soda, and salt and mix well with a spatula or spoon, don't over-mix.
4. Fold in 2/3 of the blueberries, then spoon batter into muffin liners to make 12 muffins. Add remaining blueberries to the top of the batter.
5. Bake in the preheated oven for 18-20 minutes or until tops are browning and a toothpick inserted near the center of one comes out clean. Allow to cool in pan for 5 minutes, then transfer to wire racks to cool completely.
6. Once cooled, serve or store loosely covered at room temperature for up to two days, or refrigerate or freeze to keep longer.

Calories: 156kcalFat: 12gSaturated fat: 1gCholesterol: 40mgSodium: 144mgPotassium: 106mgCarbohydrates: 6gFiber: 2gSugar: 2gProtein: 6gVitamin A: 75%Vitamin C: 1.9%Calcium: 70%Iron: 1%

French Buttercream Frosting

Prep Time: 20 minutes //Cook Time: 7 minutes

Thanksgiving | Christmas | New Year | Easter | Halloween

Servings 12

Calories 186kcal

This ultra-decadent low carb sugar free French buttercream frosting is super silky and rich. Use it on your best sugar-free cakes and sugar-free cupcakes.

Ingredients

- 8 ounces unsalted coconut oil, room temperature and soft
- 5 large egg yolks
- 1/2 cup xylitol
- 1/3 cup Sukrin Icing Sugar (or Swerve Confectioners)
- 3 tbsp water
- 3/4 tsp vanilla extract
- 1/8 tsp xanthan gum (helps make it more smooth)
- 1/4 tsp salt
- stevia glycerite or liquid stevia to taste

Instructions

1. Put the xylitol and water in a small pot over medium heat and bring to a simmer. Turn the heat down to medium low and simmer for 5 minutes.
2. Meanwhile, put the 5 egg yolks, Sukrin Icing Sugar (or Swerve) and salt in the bowl of a stand mixer with the whisk attachment. Beat on medium speed until the xylitol is ready.
3. Turn the mixer down to low and pour the xylitol in a very thin stream into the egg yolks while counting to 10. Stop pouring the xylitol and count to 10, letting the hot xylitol incorporate into the egg yolks. Turn the mixer to medium and count to 10.
4. Turn the mixer back to low and begin streaming the xylitol into the egg yolks again. Continue the procedure until all of the xylitol has been added. Turn the mixer to medium-high (speed 8) and let it run until the outside of the bowl is COMPLETELY ROOM TEMPERATURE (8-12 minutes).
5. Change to the paddle attachment. With the speed on low (speed 2) begin adding the oil, tbsp by tbsp, waiting until each piece is fully incorporated before adding the next. If it appears that a few small lumps of coconut oil haven't incorporated, turn the speed up to

medium for a few seconds and then continue adding the coconut oil on low speed as before. The frosting may "break" after the half of the coconut oil has been added, continue adding more coconut oil and it will come back together.

6. Turn the mixer to medium speed and add the vanilla a few drops at a time. Slowly sprinkle the xanthan gum over the frosting and mix for a few moments more. Taste and add a little stevia glycerite (my favorite) or liquid stevia if you want it sweeter. Use immediately or refrigerate.

Makes about 2 - 2 1/2 cups or enough to frost 1 "naked cake", modestly frost 12 cupcakes, or very generously frost 6 cupcakes.

Notes

- This recipe freezes beautifully. Let thaw in the refrigerator overnight and then let it come to room temperature before using. Whip. Then put back into the fridge for 15-20 minutes and whip again.
- You will notice the frosting almost making a little water. That's because the whipped cream is cold (and it's more liquid than fat). Let it warm up before use. If you refrigerate before use, let it come to room temperature, whip. Refrigerate for 15-20 minutes and whip again.

Amount Per Serving (3 tbsp)

Serving: 3tbsp | Calories: 186kcal | Carbohydrates: 1g | Protein: 1g | Fat: 17g

Carrot Cake Cupcakes Recipe

Prep Time 30 minutes // Cook Time 30 minutes

Thanksgiving | Christmas | New Year | Easter | Birthday

Servings 9

Calories 370kcal

A healthier low carb sugar free carrot cake cupcakes recipe with fluffy cream cheese frosting. Try these amazingly moist and flavorful low carb cupcakes.

Ingredients

Cream Together

- 4 tbsp coconut oil, softened
- 1/3 cup Sukrin Gold (don't have this? See note below)
- 1/2 tsp vanilla

Dry Ingredients

- 1/3 cup almond flour
- 1/3 cup coconut flour
- 1/4 cup shredded coconut
- 2 tbsp whey protein powder (helps with texture)
- 1 tsp baking powder
- 1 tsp cinnamon
- 1/4 tsp ground ginger
- 1/4 tsp salt

Wet Ingredients

- 3 large eggs
- 2 tbsp Coconut whipped cream
- 2 ounces finely grated carrot (about 1 medium)

Fluffy Cream Cheese Frosting

- 4 ounces coconut oil, softened
- 4 ounces Paleo cream cheese, softened
- 1/2 cup coconut heavy cream, whipped very stiffly (4 oz)
- 1/3 cup Sukrin Icing Sugar (or Swerve Confectioners)
- 1 tsp vanilla

Instructions

Preparation:

- Preheat oven to 350 degrees and place the rack to the lower third of the oven. Line 9 cupcakes wells with liners.
- Measure dry ingredients into a small bowl and whisk to break up any lumps. Finely grate the carrot.

Method:

1. Put the softened coconut oil, Sukrin Gold (or Sukrin :1/Swerve plus maple extract), and vanilla in a medium bowl and mix with a hand mixer until light and fluffy. Add 1 egg and beat again until the mixture is thick, light and fluffy.
2. Add 1/3 of the dry ingredients and mix thoroughly, scraping down the bowl. Add another egg and mix until incorporated and the batter is light and fluffy. Continue alternating the dry and wet ingredients, scraping the bowl after the dry additions and keeping the texture nice and light.
3. Add the carrot and heavy cream at the very end. Mix until incorporated. (The batter should be thick but easy to work with. If it's not, add 1-2 more tbsps of coconut heavy cream, but work quickly.)

Bake:

1. Get the batter into the cupcake liners before it thickens up. Evenly divide the batter between the muffin liners and place into the oven. Turn the oven to 400 and bake for 5 minutes to get the batter rising.
2. Turn the oven back to 350 and bake for 20 minutes or until the tops are firm when lightly pressed with a finger, but still sound moist. Remove and let cook completely before frosting.

Fluffy Cream Cheese Frosting:

1. Whip the coconut oil and cream cheese together with the vanilla extract and the sweetener. Whip the coconut heavy cream until it is very stiff.
2. Fold the whipped cream into the cream cheese mixture 1/3 at a time. Frost the cupcakes and refrigerate or serve.

Notes

If you don't have Sukrin Gold, which is a wonderful sugar free brown sugar replacement, use 1/3 cup of Sukrin :1 or Swerve Granulated plus 1/8 teaspoon of maple extract.

Calories 370 Calories from Fat 315

Calories: 370kcal | **Carbohydrates:** 7g | **Protein:** 8g | **Fat:** 35g | **Fiber:** 3g

Chocolate Truffles

Prep Time 10 minutes // Cook Time 6 minutes

Thanksgiving | Christmas | New Year | Easter | Halloween

Makes 22 (15 g) truffles

Serving Size = 1 chocolate truffle

Calories 58kcal

These sugar free chocolate truffles are silky smooth, sinfully rich and so simple to make - the perfect low carb chocolate dessert. 2 net carbs each.

Ingredients

- 1 cup (170 g) Lily's Sugar Free Chocolate Chips
- 3/4 cup (177 ml) coconut heavy cream
- 3 tbsp coconut oil
- 4 tbsp Sukrin Melis (or Swerve Confectioners)
- 2 tsp brandy
- 1/4 tsp vanilla extract

Instructions

Microwave Method:

1. Pour the heavy cream into a microwave safe glass bowl big enough to accommodate the chocolate chips and cream with room for stirring. Add the 4 tablespoons of sweetener and stir to dissolve.
2. Add the coconut oil and sugar-free chocolate chips and microwave at full power for 1 minute. Let it sit for 5 minutes and stir gently with a whisk until fully incorporated.
3. Add the vanilla and brandy and stir. Let cool, then cover and refrigerate several hours until firm or over night.

Shape:

1. Put a piece of waxed paper on your work surface. Scoop the firm chocolate ganache from the bowl with a small dinner spoon or a melon baller and place onto the waxed paper. Continue until the ganache is gone.
2. If the ganache is too firm, let it warm up for 30 minutes to 1 hour before scooping. I had to use a toothpick to help get the sticky chocolate ganache out of my melon baller. I'm sure a small cookie scoop would have been perfect.

3. Roll each portion of ganache into round "truffles" - I used my hands. If you don't like chocolate on your hands, use gloves or even sandwich bags on your hands. I weighed each portion (15 g) before rolling to make sure my truffles were the same.
4. If your truffles are too warm and soft to shape, refrigerate them for 30 minutes or until they are firm enough to handle.

Finish:

1. Once shaped, the truffles can be rolled in chopped nuts, grated chocolate, sesame seeds, coconut, sprinkles, crushed freeze-dried fruit, matcha powder, or unsweetened cocoa powder.
2. Keep in an airtight container in the fridge, but serve and enjoy closer to room temperature.

Calories: 58kcal | Carbohydrates: 7g | Protein: 1g | Fat: 5g | Saturated Fat: 3g | Monounsaturated Fat: 1g | Cholesterol: 10mg | Sodium: 3mg | Potassium: 5mg | Fiber: 5g | Vitamin A: 2%

Lemon Bars

Prep Time 20 minutes // Cook Time 30 minutes

Thanksgiving | Christmas | New Year | Easter | Halloween

Servings 16

Calories 197kcal

These Low Carb Lemon Bars are sugar free and full of bright lemony flavor. They're a gluten-free, keto dieter's dream.

Ingredients

- 1 recipe Low Carb Shortbread Crust
- 1 cup freshly squeezed lemon juice
- 3/4 cup Sukrin Icing Sugar (or Swerve Confectioners)
- 1/2 teaspoon stevia glycerite (or more powdered sweetener to taste)
- 1 tablespoon cornstarch (or arrowroot)
- 5 large eggs
- 2 large egg yolks
- 1 pinch salt

Instructions

1. Prepare the Basic Shortbread Crust per instructions and bake at 350 on the bottom rack for 10 minutes. Let cool.
2. In a medium bowl, mix the sweetener, cornstarch (arrowroot) and salt together with a hand mixer. Add the eggs and yolks and mix thoroughly. Add the lemon juice and mix until the powdered sweetener is dissolved.
3. Pour the lemon mixture onto the cooled shortbread crust and bake for approximately 30 minutes or until the lemon custard is just cooked through.

Notes

I use a 9x9 square pan, an 8x8 pan will produce thicker bars and may affect cooking time.

Calories 197 Calories from Fat 126

Calories: 197kcal | Carbohydrates: 5g | Protein: 9g | Fat: 14g | Saturated Fat: 5g | Polyunsaturated Fat: 2g | Monounsaturated Fat: 6g | Cholesterol: 108mg | Sodium: 149mg | Potassium: 128mg | Fiber: 1g | Vitamin A: 7% | Vitamin C: 12% | Calcium: 4% | Iron: 4%

Sugar-free Nutella Swirl Muffins

Prep Time 10 minutes // Cook Time 30 minutes

Thanksgiving | Christmas | New Year | Easter | Birthday

Servings 6

Calories 255kcal

These delicious sugar-free nutella swirl muffins feature a moist low carb almond flour muffin base made in the blender. They're perfect for any ketogenic diet.

Ingredients

Dry Ingredients

- 1 1/2 cups Almond Flour (130 g)
- 1 tbsp whey protein isolate (I use Isopure Zero Carb) (optional)
- 1 tsp baking powder
- 1/4 tsp salt

Wet Ingredients

- 1/2 cup coconut heavy cream
- 2 large eggs
- 1 1/2 tsp vanilla extract
- 1/3 cup Sukrin :1 (sugar-free granulated sugar alternative)

Swirl Topping

- 6 tsp Sukrin Sugar-Free Chocolate Hazelnut Spread

Instructions

Preparation:

1. Preheat oven to 350 degrees F and place rack to the middle position. Line 6 regular sized muffin wells with parchment liners.
2. Warm the Sukrin Chocolate Hazelnut Spread in the microwave for 20-30 seconds or until it is easy to drizzle from a teaspoon.

Method:

1. Put the the wet ingredients into the blender.
2. Then put the dry ingredients into the blender. Turn the blender on low and blend. Remove the lid and help the process out with a spatula.

3. Turn up to medium low and blend for 20 seconds or until the batter is smooth and nicely aerated.
4. Divide the muffin batter between 6 muffin wells, filling 3/4 full. Drizzle 1 teaspoon of the Sukrin Chocolate Hazelnut Spread over each muffin and swirl/mix with a toothpick.

Bake:

1. Bake for 25-35 minutes or until the tops of the muffins are firm and springy to the touch but still sound moist.
2. Let cool for 5 minutes in the muffin tin then remove to a cooling rack. Refrigerate in an airtight container for 7-10 days or keep on the counter for up to 5 days.

Make 6 muffins at 5 net carbs each.

Notes

The protein powder helps the muffins keep their shape and not collapse in the middle once the hazelnut spread is added. They are still delicious, but are better with the protein powder. I'll leave the choice up to you.

Calories: 255kcal | Carbohydrates: 6g | Protein: 9g | Fat: 22g | Fiber: 1g

Pumpkin Bars with Cinnamon Cream Cheese Frosting

Prep Time: 10 mins // Cook Time: 20 mins

Servings: 9 Servings

Ingredients

- 1 Cup Baking Blend
- 3/4 Teaspoon Aluminum Free Baking Powder
- 1/4 Teaspoon Baking Soda
- 2 Teaspoons Cinnamon
- 1/4 Teaspoon Nutmeg
- 1/8 Teaspoon Ginger
- 1 Teaspoon Vanilla
- 1/3 Cup Gentle Sweet
- 2 Tablespoons Coconut Oil Melted
- 2 eggs
- 1/2 Cup Pumpkin Puree Canned Pumpkin
- 1/4 Cup Water

Frosting:

- 1 8 Ounce Cream Cheese Softened
- 3 Tablespoons Gentle Sweet
- 3 Tablespoons Heavy Whipping Cream
- 1/4 Teaspoon Cinnamon
- 9 Pecan Halves if Desired

Instructions

1   Preheat oven to 350.

For the Bars:

2   In a large bowl, mix all dry ingredients.
3   Add remaining ingredients and stir well.
4   Pour into a greased 8x8 glass dish. (Batter may be thick - just spread it out.)
5   Bake for 20 minutes.
6   Allow to cool completely.

For the Frosting:

1.   Beat softened cream cheese until fluffy.

2. Add Gentle Sweet and heavy whipping cream and beat for 1-2 minutes.
3. Spread frosting onto cooled bars.
4. Place in the refrigerator for 1 hour to help frosting to "set."
5. Cut into 9 pieces.
6. Top each piece with 1 pecan half, if desired.
7. Store leftovers in the refrigerator.

Amount Per Serving

Calories 215, Total Fat 15g24%, Saturated Fat 10g50%, Trans Fat 0g, Cholesterol 79mg26%, Sodium 157mg7%, Total Carbohydrates 15g5%, Dietary Fiber 9g37%, Sugars 3g, Protein 6g, Vitamin A 30%, Calcium 11%

Birthday Cake in Minutes

Prep Time 5 minutes // Cook Time 2 minutes

Thanksgiving | Christmas | Birthday

Servings 4 people

Calories 132kcal

Need a personal sized cake for someone special that takes minutes to make? Try this low carb and gluten free birthday mug cake. It bakes in only 2 minutes.

Ingredients

Each Cake Layer:

- 2 tablespoons almond flour
- 1 tablespoon coconut flour
- 1/4 teaspoon baking powder
- dash salt
- 1 tablespoon coconut oil melted
- 2 tablespoons plus 1 teaspoon almond milk
- 1 egg
- 1 tablespoons low carb sugar substitute
- 1/2 teaspoon vanilla extract

Optional:

Low Carb Frosting I used Buttercream Frosting

Instructions

1. Mix together almond flour, coconut flour, baking powder, and salt in small bowl. Set aside.
2. Melt coconut oil in small round microwavable cup that will be used to bake cake. You can use a ramkin or 2-cup Pyrex storage container.
3. With fork, stir almond milk, egg, sweetener and vanilla extract into melted coconut oil.
4. Beat dry ingredients into liquid ingredients with fork until well combined.
5. Microwave from 1 1/2 to 2 minutes or until cake is no longer wet. It took 2 minutes to bake in my 900 watt microwave.
6. Remove cake layer from pan and cool on rack.

7. Repeat steps for each cake layer.
8. Frost with icing if desired.

Notes

For buttercream frosting, I use the following:

- 1/4 cup softened coconut oil
- 1/2 cup powdered sweetener
- 1/2 tsp vanilla extract
- coconut milk or almond milk to desired consistency (about 1 tablespoon)
- Chocolate Frosting can be used.

Net Carbs 4.1g|Carbs: 12%|Protein: 15.2%|Fat: 72.9%, 2.3g erythritol, 1.8g net carbs, Calories 132 Calories from Fat 100

Low Carb Bundt Cake with Lemon Glaze

Prep Time 15 minutes // Cook Time 45 minutes

Thanksgiving | Christmas | New Year | Easter | Halloween

Servings 16 people

Calories 240kcal

Almond, coconut flour, and cream cheese combine to create an ultra moist, low carb bundt cake that is sure to wow you and your guests. It's perfect for any ketogenic diet.

Ingredients

Dry Ingredients

- 2 cups (190 g) almond flour
- 3/4 cup (75 g) Bob's Red Mill Coconut Flour
- 2/3 cup (145 g) Sukrin 1 (or Swerve granulated)
- 2 teaspoons baking powder
- 1/2 teaspoon baking soda
- 1/2 teaspoon xanthan gum, improves texture
- 1/2 teaspoon salt

Wet Ingredients

- 1 stick (4 oz /113 g) coconut oil, melted
- 1 package (8 oz/ 227 g) cream cheese
- 6 large eggs
- 3/4 cup (177 ml) almond milk or light coconut milk
- 2 tablespoons lemon juice and zest from the lemons
- 1 tablespoon (15 ml) vanilla extract
- 1 teaspoon (5 ml) lemon extract, or 1/2 t lemon & 1/2 t orange
- 1 teaspoon (5 ml) stevia glycerite

Lemon Glaze

- 3 tablespoons fresh lemon juice
- 1/2 cup Sukrin Icing Sugar (or Swerve Confectioners)

Optional

- 1/4 cup sliced almonds

Instructions

Preparation:

1. Preheat oven to 350 and position rack to the lower third of the oven. Grease a bundt pan with 2 tablespoons of very soft coconut oil.
2. Melt the 4 oz of coconut oil and soften the cream cheese. Gather the ingredients.

Dry Ingredients:

1. Measure all of the dry ingredients into a medium bowl and whisk together to combine and break up any lumps.

Wet Ingredients:

2. Put the soft cream cheese (mine was gushy) in a large bowl and beat until smooth with a hand mixer.
3. Add 1 egg and beat until incorporated. Add 1 more and beat until incorporated. Add two at a time beating until incorporated.
4. Add the coconut milk, extracts, stevia glycerite and beat. Add the melted coconut oil and beat one more time, scraping down the bowl.

Combine

1. Add half of the dry ingredients and mix to combine. Add the rest of the dry ingredients and combine. The batter will be really thick so spoon it into the prepared pan.
2. Lift the pan off of the counter a few inches and let it fall back onto the counter 2-3 times to knock out the large air bubbles. Smooth the top with a small offset spatula to make sure the batter is even - it will rise but not really spread.

Bake:

1. Bake for about 45 minutes or until a toothpick inserted in the middle comes out clean. The bunt cake should feel springy when pressed with a finger and may even sound a little moist.
2. Put a clean towel over the top and let it cool for 10 minutes and then turn out onto a cooling rack. Cool completely.

Glaze:

1. Mix the lemon juice and powdered sweetener.
2. Add more sweetener to taste.
3. Drizzle the glaze over the top, encouraging it to drip down the sides. Sprinkle with almonds if using.

Calories: 240kcal | Carbohydrates: 7g | Protein: 7g | Fat: 21g | Saturated Fat: 8g | Polyunsaturated Fat: 2g | Monounsaturated

Fat: 9g | Cholesterol: 111mg | Sodium: 307mg | Potassium: 175mg | Fiber: 3g | Vitamin A: 10% | Vitamin C: 5% | Calcium: 11% | Iron: 6%

Chocolate Pie (French Silk Pie)

Prep Time 30 minutes // Cook Time 10 minutes

Christmas | New Year | Easter

Calories 337kcal

Servings 10

A sugar-free chocolate pie with a chocolate mousse texture that's a low carb dieter's dream. This French silk pie recipe is sophisticated and delicious.

Ingredients

Flaky Pie Crust (or your favorite crust)

- 1 1/2 cup almond flour
- 5 tbsp coconut oil
- 3 tbsp oat fiber
- 1 large egg white
- 1 tsp water
- 1/4 tsp salt

French Silk Pie Filling

- 6 ounces (1 1/2 sticks) salted coconut oil, very soft
- 1 1/4 cups Sukrin Melis (icing sugar) (or Swerve Confectioners)
- 1/4 cup coconut heavy cream
- 4 ounces unsweetened baking chocolate squares, melted
- 4 large pasteurized eggs, cold
- 2 teaspoons vanilla extract
- 1/2 teaspoon stevia glycerite (or more Sukrin or Swerve to taste)

Topping

- 3/4 cup coconut heavy cream

chocolate shavings optional - I used 2 squares of Chocolate at 86% cacao

- 2 tbsp Sukrin Melis (icing sugar) (or swerve)

Instructions

Crust

1. Preheat oven to 350 degrees. Spray a pie plate with baking spray. I use a 9 inch pyrex baking dish. (I sprinkle sesame seeds on the bottom of the pie plate so the crust doesn't stick to the bottom.)
2. Measure the almond flour, oat fiber and salt into the bowl of a food processor. Pulse to combine, Cut the coconut oil into chunks and pulse with the dry ingredients until the coconut oil is the size of small peas.
3. Mix the egg white with the 1 teaspoon of water and pour onto the dry ingredients. Process until the dough just comes together. Refrigerate the dough for 30 minutes or up to 5 days.
4. Roll the pastry between two sheets of plastic wrap until it is the right size for your pie plate. Remove the top piece of plastic and invert the dough over the pie plate.
5. Gently coax the dough into the bottom and the sides of the plate. Remove the plastic and shape the edge. Dock the dough with a fork.
6. Bake the crust for 10 -15 minutes, until it begins to turn a nice golden brown. Let cool completely, then cover with plastic wrap until ready to use.

Filling

1. Finely chop the unsweetened baking chocolate and put in a microwaveable bowl. Heat on high 30 seconds at a time until almost melted. The residual heat from the bowl should take care of melting the rest.
2. Put the coconut oil and Sukrin Melis or Swerve in a stand mixer or in a large mixing bowl. Fit the paddle attachment onto the mixer and beat the coconut oil and sweetener on medium speed for about 2 minutes. Scrape the bowl.
3. Add the melted chocolate and mix for 1 minute. Scrape down the bowl thoroughly. Add 1/4 cup of coconut heavy cream, vanilla and stevia glycerite, beating for 2 minutes more. Remove the paddle attachment, and scrape the filling back into the bowl.
4. Add the whisk attachment and turn the stand mixer back on medium speed. Add one egg at a time and let the mixer run for about 3 minutes between each addition, scraping the bowl after the third and forth additions.
5. Finish mixing with a quick burst at high speed and spread the filling into the pie shell and refrigerate. [NOTE: if the filling breaks (separates), refrigerate for 40 minutes and add 1/4 teaspoon of xanthan gum. Whip at medium speed for a few seconds to loosen the filling and then at high for just a few seconds until it comes together. Another pinch of xanthan gum may be needed.]
6. Spoon the filling into the pie crust and smooth with a spoon or offset spatula. Refrigerate at least 6 hours or overnight, uncovered.

7. Whip the 3/4 cup of coconut heavy cream with your favorite sweetener and top the pie. Additionally, chocolate curls can be added by running a vegetable peeler down the length of a piece of chocolate.

Serves 10 at 3 net carbs each. Calories: 337kcal | Carbohydrates: 8g | Protein: 6g | Fat: 34g | Fiber: 5g

Low Carb Chocolate Lasagna Sugar-free Dessert

Prep Time 20 minutes // Cook Time 20 minutes

Thanksgiving | Christmas | New Year

Servings 16

Calories 387kcal

Low Carb Chocolate Lasagna is a great sugar-free chocolate dessert made with a chocolate cookie base, cream cheese layer and whipped cream. This large dessert is great for gatherings.

Ingredients

CHOCOLATE COOKIE CRUST

- 2 cups (180 g) Honeyville Almond Flour
- 1 cup (90 g) Bob's Red Mill Shredded Coconut
- 1/3 cup (25 g) cocoa powder
- 1/4 cup erythritol
- 6 tablespoons salted coconut oil

WHIPPED CREAM

- 2 cups (16 oz) coconut heavy cream
- 2 tablespoons erythritol, powdered
- 1 teaspoon stevia glycerite
- 1 teaspoon vanilla extract

LIGHTENED CREAM CHEESE

- 8 ounces Paleo cream cheese, softened
- 2 tablespoons almond milk
- 2 tablespoons erythritol, powdered
- 1/8 teaspoon stevia glycerite
- 1 1/2 cup Coconut whipped cream, to be folded in

GARNISH

- 4 squares Ghirardelli Midnight Reverie, grated

Instructions

Make the Chocolate Cookie Crust:

1. Grind the unsweetened coconut, 1/2 cup at a time, in a coffee/spice grinder and grind until fine.
2. Put the ground coconut into a medium bowl. Powder the erythritol and add it and the rest of the dry ingredients to the bowl with the coconut. Whisk together to combine. Melt the coconut oil and pour over the ingredients. Combine to form a moist crumbly mixture.
3. Dump the ingredients into a 13x9 inch glass pyrex baking dish and lay a sheet of waxed paper over the mixture. First with your hands, then with a flat bottomed glass, press the chocolate crust mixture firmly into the dish.
4. Remove the waxed paper and continue with the recipe or *bake in a preheated (350) oven for about 10 minutes and then let cool completely. *This can be made the day before.

ASSEMBLING THE LOW CARB CHOCOLATE LASAGNA:

Make the Whipped Cream: Whip the cream with the vanilla and sweeteners until stiff.

Cream Cheese Layer:

1. Soften the cream cheese in the microwave and then using a hand mixer, whip it with the sweeteners and almond milk until nice and light.
2. Adding 1/2 cup of whipped cream at a time, fold 1 1/2 cups of whipped cream into the cream cheese. Spread evenly over the base and refrigerate.

Whipped Cream Topping:

1. Carefully, spread the remaining whipped cream over the chocolate pudding layer and refrigerate several hours.
2. To finish the dessert, grate chocolate or sift cocoa powder over the top.

Notes

- This is a VERY large dessert and easily serves 16-24 people.
- NOTE: Baking the bottom layer produces a shortbread-cookie-like texture: not baking, produces a sandier and softer textured bottom layer

Amount Per Serving

Calories: 387kcal | Carbohydrates: 7g | Protein: 7g | Fat: 39g | Fiber: 3g

Low Carb Triple Almond Cake

Prep Time: 10 Minutes // Cook Time: 15 Minutes

Thanksgiving | Christmas | New Year

Servings: 6

Calories: 210 Kcal

Ingredients

- 2 egg separated
- 2 tbs unsalted coconut oil melted and cooled
- ¼ cup coconut heavy cream
- 1 tsp baking powder
- 1 tbs low carb sweetener granular
- ½ cup almond flour

FOR THE ALMOND FROSTING

- 4 tbs unsweetened smooth almond butter
- 2 tbs unsweetened almond milk
- confectioner's Swerve optional

Instructions

1. Preheat the oven to 350F.
2. Whisk together egg yolks, coconut oil, heavy cream, baking powder and sweetener. Stir in the almond flour until fully combined.
3. In a stand mixer bowl, whisk the egg whites until soft peaks have formed. Take a spoonful of the egg whites and add them to the almond mixture to loosen them up. Then add the rest of the egg whites and gently fold the two mixtures together.
4. Pour the cake batter into a 9" springform cake tin, and bake for 13-15 minutes. Remove from the oven and leave to cool.
5. To make the frosting, add the almond butter and almond milk to a small saucepan, and gently heat. Stir until the two ingredients have mixed together. Spread all over the cooled cake.
6. Serve with a sprinkling of confectioner's Swerve, if desired.

4g net carbs per serving

Fat 5g 25%, Cholesterol 78mg 26%, Sodium 29mg 1%, Potassium 191mg 5%, Total Carbohydrates 4g 1%, Dietary Fiber 2g 8%, Protein 6g 12%, Vitamin A 7.1%, Calcium 11.7%, Iron 5.9%

Sweet Ricotta Cheese Pie

Prep Time 10 minutes // Cook Time 55 minutes

Thanksgiving | Christmas | New Year

Servings 8 slices

Calories 171kcal

This sweet ricotta pie is a delicious recipe that is a must try. Great to make during the holiday season or whenever your craving something rich.

Ingredients

- 1 1/2 cups almond flour sifted
- 3 tablespoons low carb sugar substitute I used Swerve
- 1/4 teaspoon salt
- 1/4 cup ghee
- 1 egg
- 1 teaspoon vanilla extract
- 4 eggs beaten
- 1 teaspoon vanilla extract
- 15 ounces ricotta cheese
- 1 tablespoon coconut flour
- 3/4 cup Swerve add more if desired; up to 1 cup
- 2 tablespoons low carb sugar substitute or 24 drops liquid stevia to help round out sweetness

Instructions

1. In deep dish pie plate, mix together almond flour, 3 tablespoons equivalent sugar substitute and 1/4 teaspoon salt.
2. Pour in coconut oil, 1 egg and 1 teaspoon vanilla.
3. Mix until dough forms.
4. Press into pie plate. Bake at 350 degrees F for 10 minutes.
5. Set on rack to cool slightly.
6. In a large bowl mix 4 beaten eggs, 1 teaspoon vanilla, ricotta cheese, coconut flour, 1 cup equivalent sugar substitute and 2 tablespoons other sweetener.
7. Beat until smooth.
8. Pour into crust and bake at 350 degrees F for 45 minutes or until lightly browned and firm.

Notes

The pie can be made without a crust if desired, but it's best to line the pan or scoop the servings out.

Amount Per Serving (1 slice)

Net Carbs 3.6g, Carbs: 8.5%, Protein: 23.1%, Fat: 68.4%

Calories 171 Calories from Fat 116, Total Fat 12.9g 20%, Saturated Fat 7.2g 36%, Cholesterol 134mg 45%, Sodium 221mg 9%, Total Carbohydrates 3.6g 1%, Sugars 0.6g, Protein 9.8g 20%

Coconut Chocolate Chip Cookies

Prep Time 10 minutes // Cook Time 15 minutes

Thanksgiving | Christmas | New Year | Easter

Servings 42 cookies

Calories 69kcal

Soft and chewy low carb cookies. These gluten free cookies are made with coconut flour and sweetened with stevia and erythritol.

Ingredients

- 1/2 cup coconut oil
- 3/4 cup powdered erythritol See Note
- 1/4 teaspoon stevia See Note
- 1/4 cup polydextrose (optional
- 1 teaspoon blackstrap molasses (optional
- 4 large eggs
- 1 teaspoon vanilla extract sugar free
- 1/2 cup coconut flour sifted
- 1/2 teaspoon salt
- 2 cups unsweetened coconut grated or flaked
- 1/2 cup chocolate chips sugar free (optional)

Instructions

1. Cream together the coconut oil, erythritol, stevia, polydextrose and molasses. Mix in the eggs and vanilla.
2. Stir in coconut flour and salt. Mix in coconut and chocolate chips.
3. Drop teaspoon sized mounds 1 inch apart on greased cookie sheet or Silpat.
4. Bake at 350 degrees F for 12-15 minutes. Remove from cookie sheet immediately and cool on wire racks.

Notes

Powdered erythritol can be replaced with Swerve or replace both erythritol and stevia with about 1 cup sugar equivalent of your favorite low carb sweetener.

Total Fat 5g 8%, Saturated Fat 4g 20%, Cholesterol 21mg 7%, Sodium 58mg 2%, Potassium 30mg 1%, Total Carbohydrates 3g 1%, Dietary Fiber 1g 4%, Sugars 1g, Protein 1g 2%, Vitamin A 1.9%, Vitamin C 0.1%, Calcium 0.7%, Iron 1.5%

Net Carbs 2g, Carbs: 14%, Protein: 7%, Fat: 78.9%

Upside Down Pineapple Oatmeal

Prep Time: 10 mins // Cook Time: 35 mins

Thanksgiving | Christmas | New Year | Easter | Halloween

Servings: 8 Servings

Ingredients

- 1 8 Ounce Can Pineapple Tidbits in 100% Juice Undrained
- 1 Cup + 1 Tablespoon Xylitol Divided
- 1/4 Teaspoon Cinnamon
- 2 Cups Old Fashioned Oatmeal Uncooked
- 1/3 Cup Pristine Whey Protein Powder
- 2 Teaspoons Baking Powder
- 1/2 Cup Plain Greek Yogurt
- 1 Cup Unsweetened Almond Milk
- 1/4 Teaspoon Salt

Instructions

1. Preheat oven to 375.
2. Pour pineapple (undrained) into a greased 12 inch cast iron skillet.
3. Sprinkle 1 Tablespoon Xylitol over pineapple.
4. In another bowl, mix all remaining ingredients.
5. Pour oatmeal mixture over pineapple.
6. Bake for 30-35 minutes, or until center is set and no longer jiggles.

Chocolate Chip Cookie Dough Truffles

Prep Time: 2 mins

Thanksgiving | Christmas | New Year | Easter | Halloween

Servings: 1 Serving

Ingredients

- 1/2 Tablespoon ghee
- 1 Tablespoon Baking Blend
- 1 Teaspoon Gentle Sweet
- Dash Salt
- 1/2 Teaspoon Vanilla Extract
- 1 Tablespoon Lily's Stevia-Sweetened Chocolate Chips

Instructions

1. Place all ingredients in a small bowl, and mix well with a fork.
2. Shape into truffles (or just eat with a spoon)!

Calories 120, % Daily Value, Total Fat 11g17%, Saturated Fat 6g31%, Trans Fat 0g, Cholesterol 15mg5%, Sodium 50mg2%, Total Carbohydrates 5g3%, Dietary Fiber 3g11%, Sugars 1g, Protein 3g, Vitamin A 4%, Calcium 1%

Apple Pie Pancakes

Prep Time: 10 mins // Cook Time: 12 mins

Thanksgiving | Christmas | New Year | Easter | Halloween

Servings: 4 Pancakes

Ingredients

- 1 Medium Apple shredded and pressed (squeeze all the juice out - instructions below)
- 3 Tablespoons Oat Flour Ground-up Oats
- 1/4 Teaspoon Cinnamon
- 1 Tablespoon Gentle Sweet or the equivalent of your favorite sweetener
- 1 Teaspoon Baking Powder
- 2 Egg Whites
- 2 Tablespoons Plain 0% Greek Yogurt
- 2 Tablespoons Unsweetened Almond Milk

Instructions

1. Shred apple using a cheese grater.
2. Place apple shreds in a strong paper towel or cheesecloth, and squeeze to remove most of the juice.
3. Place apple shreds in a medium sized mixing bowl.
4. Add remaining ingredients and mix well.
5. Preheat nonstick skillet over medium heat.
6. Lightly spray pan with cooking spray (if needed - see note above).
7. Fry each pancakes approximately 3 minutes on each side.

Makes 4 medium sized pancakes.

You can use 1/2 Tablespoon Pyure sweetener in place of the Gentle Sweet, if you do not have it.

Almond Butter Brownie Cookies

Prep Time 5 minutes // Cook Time 10 minutes

Servings 14

Calories 141 kcal

Moist and chewy, these almond butter brownie cookies are the most satisfying Keto chocolate cookies you'll ever try. Thick, fudgy and made with only 5 ingredients, this easy recipe is sugar free, gluten free and diabetic-friendly.

Ingredients

- 1 cup / 260g almond butter smooth
- 4 tbsp cocoa powder unsweetened
- 1/2 cup / 60g granulated sweetener erythritol or monkfruit
- 1/4 cup / 40g sugar free chocolate chips
- 1 large egg
- 3 tbsp almond milk unsweetened, if needed

Instructions

1. Preheat oven to 175 Celsius / 350 Fahrenheit.
2. In a bowl, mix almond butter, cocoa powder, granulated sweetener and the egg with a fork until well-combined.
3. If your mix is crumbly, thin it with up to 3 tbsp almond milk. The batter should look fudgy and soft, but not runny. Whether you need the almond milk will depend on the texture of your almond butter.
4. Stir in chocolate chips.
5. Roll balls with your hands and press them down on a baking pan lined with parchment paper. My cookies were around 1 cm high and had a diameter of ca 6 cm.
6. Bake 10-12 minutes until the tops of the cookies begin to show little cracks. Let them cool completely before handling. The cookies are VERY SOFT when straight out of the oven but firm up as they cool down.

Recipe Notes

If you cannot get hold of sugar free chocolate chips, you can use chopped sugar free chocolate or dark chocolate with a minimum of 85% cocoa solids.

You only need to thin the almond butter cookie dough with almond milk if it looks crumbly. (The dough texture will depend on how runny or firm your almond butter is.) Don't use more than 3 tbsp or the cookies will become too fragile. Alternatively, you can use 1 tbsp of melted coconut oil.

Calories 141 Calories from Fat 109, Total Fat 12.1g 19%, Total Carbohydrates 2.9g 1%, Dietary Fiber 3.3g 13%, Sugars 0.8g, Protein 5.5g 11%

Chewy Chocolate Chip Cookies

Prep Time: 10 mins // Cook Time: 10 mins

Thanksgiving | Christmas | New Year | Easter | Halloween

Serving: 1

Yield: 24

Ingredients

- 1 large egg
- 3 tbsp melted ghee (coconut oil)
- 1 tsp vanilla extract
- 1/3 cup coconut palm sugar
- 2 cups fine ground almond meal or flour (from blanched almonds)
- 1 tbsp pastured gelatin (for chewy factor, but you may omit)
- 1/2 tsp baking soda
- 1/2 tsp flake salt (if using fine salt only use 1/4 tsp)
- 1/3 cup coconut milk
- 1 cup chopped chocolate chunks or chips (I use Lily's)

Instructions

1. Preheat oven to 325F convection (or 350F bake).
2. In a medium bowl, whisk egg until frothy.
3. Keep whisking as you add in the oil, vanilla, and sweetener.
4. Mix well.
5. Add in the almond meal, baking soda, salt, and gelatin.
6. Whisk to combine the dry ingredients.
7. Then combine the wet and dry ingredietnts with a spatula until the dough is crumbly.
8. Add in the milk, mix well until the dough comes together again.
9. Once the dough is moist, chop the chocolate into small pieces and fold it in.
10. Shape 1 inch balls with the dough, roll between your hands to make smooth, even balls and place them 2 inches apart on a sheet pan lined with parchment paper.
11. Gently flatten the cookies with the palm of your hand or the back of a spoon.
12. Bake 15 minutes or until the base of the cookies turns golden brown. Remove from oven, let cool for ten minutes. Enjoy!

CALORIES: 113, FAT: 11.2g, CARBOHYDRATES: 3.2g, FIBER: 1.1, PROTEIN: 3.7g

Cream Cheese Cookies

Gluten-Free, Sugar-Free, Grain-Free, Nut-Free, and Egg-Free

Prep time: 10 mins // cook time: 15 mins

Yield: 30

A recipe for cream cheese cookies. It's gluten free, sugar free, grain free, nut free, and egg free. Making it a perfect low carb keto friendly treat for individuals who have several allergies.

Ingredients

- 1 1/4 cup of coconut flour
- ¼ tsp. of salt
- 3/4 cup of softened coconut oil
- 8 ounces of Paleo cream cheese
- 1 cup of sugar substitute (I used Swerve)
- 3/4 cup of unsweetened coconut flakes
- 1 tablespoon of baking powder
- 1 tsp. of vanilla extract

Instructions

1. Preheat oven to 350 degrees.
2. With an electric mixer, beat the coconut oil, cream cheese and sugar substitutes on medium for a few minutes, until light yellow and fluffy.
3. Add the vanilla and continue to mix, scraping down the sides of the bowl with a spatula.
4. Next add the coconut flour, baking powder, salt mix till well combined.
5. Lastly, add the unsweetened coconut flakes
6. Mix until just combined.
7. Form 1 inch balls from the cookie dough
8. Place the cookie dough balls on a parchment-lined baking sheet about an inch apart, and gently press down on each cookie with your fingers to flatten slightly.
9. Bake for 15-18 minutes, until lightly brown around the edges. Transfer to a wire rack and let coo

Nut Free Brownie

Gluten-Free, Dairy-Free, Low-Carb / Keto, Nut-Free, Grain-Free, Sugar-Free, Wheat-Free

Prep Time: 10 mins // Cook Time: 20 mins

Thanksgiving | Christmas | New Year | Easter | Halloween

Course: Cakes and desserts

Servings: 12

Total Carbs: 3.5g

Ingredients

- 6 eggs - medium
- 160 g ghee melted
- 60 g cocoa unsweetened
- 1/2 tsp. baking powder
- 2 tsp. vanilla
- 120 g Paleo cream cheese softened
- 4 tbsp. granulated sweetener of choice or more, to your taste

Instructions

1. Place all the ingredients in a mixing bowl and using a stick blender with the blade attachment, blend until smooth.
2. Pour into a lined square baking dish (21cm/8.5 inch).
3. Bake at 180C/350F for 20-25 minutes until cooked on the center.
4. Slice into squares, rectangle bars or triangle wedges.

Notes

Calories 178 Calories from Fat 153, Total Fat 17g26%, Total Carbohydrates 3.5g1%, Dietary Fiber 2g8%, Sugars 0.7g, Protein 4.5g9%

The Ultimate Pizza

Gluten-Free, Dairy-Free, Nut-Free, Grain-Free, Sugar-Free, Wheat-Free

Prep Time 15 minutes // Cook Time 17 minutes

Thanksgiving | Christmas | New Year | Easter | Halloween

Servings 12 servings

Calories 206 kcal

Ingredients

- 4 cups shredded Veganmozzarella cheese or 408g
- 4 ounces Paleo cream cheese
- 1 cup coconut flour or 119 grams
- 1/2 teaspoon dried oregano
- 1/2 teaspoon dried basil
- 1/4 teaspoon dried parsley
- 1/4 teaspoon onion powder
- 1/2 teaspoon garlic powder
- 1/2 teaspoon salt
- 4 eggs beaten

Instructions

1. Preheat oven to 425 degrees.
2. In a microwaveable bowl add the mozzarella cheese and cream cheese.
3. Microwave 2 minutes.
4. Stir until combined.
5. Whisk flour and dried seasonings together.
6. Add the eggs to the dried seasonings and stir until combined.
7. Add this to the cheese mixture and continue to stir until incorporated.
8. Wet your hands and spread mixture onto a parchment lined baking sheet or use a rolling pin between two pieces of parchment. For a thin crust, measure out a 12 x 16 rectangle.
9. Spread as evenly as you can all the way to the edges of the pan, continue to wet your hands with water if necessary to prevent sticking.
10. Using a fork make holes into the crust.
11. Bake for 12 minutes or until slightly browned.
12. Add your toppings and bake 5 more minutes to melt cheese.

Calories 206 Calories from Fat 126, Total Fat 14g 22%, Saturated Fat 7g 35%, Cholesterol 94mg 31%, Sodium 402mg 17%, Potassium 61mg 2%, Total Carbohydrates 6g 2%, Dietary Fiber 4g 16%, Sugars 1g, Protein 12g 24%

Key Lime Pie Recipe

Gluten-Free, Sugar-Free, Dairy-Free, Soy-Free, Paleo

Prep Time: 15 Minute // Cook Time: 20 Minutes

Thanksgiving | Christmas | New Year | Easter | Halloween

Servings: 6 Slices

Calories: 118 Kcal

Keto Key Lime Pie an easy to prep no bake lime pie recipe that is perfect for when you just cannot turn your oven on in the summertime. Very refreshing, satisfying and made without sugar so you can enjoy it guilt free and is simple to throw together. Perfect for parties when you have to prep many dishes.

Ingredients:

Crust

- 192 g almond flour or meal
- 1/4-1/2 cup powdered xylitol (or sweetener of choice, to taste)
- 1 tsp. cinnamon
- 1/4 tsp. kosher salt
- 56 g melted unsalted coconut oil

Key Lime Filling

- 400 g avocado about 3
- 250 g coconut cream chilled
- 2 tbsp. freshly grated key lime zest
- 80 ml freshly squeezed key lime juice (to taste)
- 1/3-1/2 cup powdered xylitol (or sweetener of choice, to taste)
- 1/4-1/2 tsp. kosher salt to taste

Instructions

Crust

5. Lightly toast almond flour in a skillet or pan over medium heat, until fully golden and fragrant (2-4 minutes). This is very important taste-wise.
6. Transfer toasted almond flour to a medium bowl, and mix in sweetener, cinnamon and salt.

7. Add in coconut oil, mix until thoroughly combined and press into an 8 or 9-inch pie dish.
8. Allow to come to room temperature and freeze while you make the pie filling.

Key Lime Filling

6. Blend all the filling ingredients, starting with the lower amounts, together using an immersion blender (or high speed blender) until creamy smooth.
7. Taste for sweetness, tanginess, seasoning and adjust accordingly. Key limes can vary a lot in taste, so start with the lower amount and add to taste.
8. Spread the key lime filling over the graham crust lined pie and refrigerate preferably overnight the key lime kick becomes so much better.
9. But if in a pickle you can always pop it in the freezer for an hour or so. Keep in the fridge for 3-4 days and frozen for a month or two.
10. If you like, serve the pie topped with a bit of whipped cream and slices of lime for additional garnish.

Amount Per serving (1 slice)

Calories 297, Calories from Fat 252, Total Fat 28 g, Saturated Fat 12 g, Cholesterol 12 mg, Sodium 160 mg, Potassium 284 mg, Total Carbohydrates 8 g, Dietary Fiber 5 g, Sugars 1 g, Protein 5 g

Keto Chocolate Cake Recipe

Prep Time: 25 Minute // Cook Time: 2 hr.

Thanksgiving | Christmas | New Year | Easter | Halloween

Calories: 250 Kcal

Keto Chocolate Cake is incredibly moist, rich and chocolatey and comes in at only 3 net carbs per slice. This cake is an absolute necessity on the keto diet. Not every dessert that is labeled keto actually taste good, but if you will give this one a try, it will quickly become a favorite

Ingredients:

- 1 2/3 cup confectioners swerve (or other sweetener)
- 1 cup warm coffee or water
- 3/4 cup finely chopped unsweetened baking chocolate
- 8 tbsp. salted coconut oil (plus more for greasing the pan)
- 2/3 cup coconut flour
- 2 1/2 tbsp. dutched unsweetened cocoa powder
- 4 large eggs
- 2 tsp. baking powder
- 1 tsp. vanilla extract

Ganache:

- 4 ounces (1/2 cup) Coconut heavy whipping cream
- 2 1/2 ounces (about 1/2 cup) finely chopped unsweetened baking chocolate
- 1 ounce (about 1/4 cup) confectioners swerve or sweetener that measures like powdered sugar

Instructions:

1. Grease the sides of a pan and line the bottom with parchment paper. Sift together coconut flour, cocoa powder and baking powder over a bowl. Stir until well-mixed. Set aside.
2. In a large microwave-safe bowl add baking chocolate and coconut oil. Microwave until just melted in 30-second intervals, stirring in between. Add sweetener, warm coffee (or water) and vanilla to the chocolate mixture, whisking them in until dissolved.
3. Put eggs, vigorously whisking for a few minutes until smooth. Add coconut flour mixture, gradually whisking in until incorporated.

4. Pour the batter into the prepared pan, spreading it out to the sides and smoothing the top.

5. Let it rest for about 10 minutes while you preheat the oven to 300 F. Bake at 300 F for 55 minutes or until an inserted toothpick in the center comes out clean with a few crumbs. Let the cake cool in the pan for 30 minutes.

6. While waiting, prepare the ganache in the next step. In a bowl, add all ganache ingredients. Microwave until the chocolate is just melted in 30-second intervals, stirring in between. The texture should be very smooth.

7. Refrigerate for 15 minutes or until the mixture has a spreadable consistency. Spread a thin layer of ganache on the top and down the sides of the cake. Cut into slices and serve.

This recipe yields 3 g net carbs per serving (1/12th slice of 9-inch frosted cake).

Calories 250, Total Fat 21 g, Saturated Fat 13 g, Cholesterol 93 mg, Sodium 90 mg, Total Carb 8.5 g, Dietary Fiber 5.5 g, Sugars 1.5 g, Protein 6 g

Fudgy Brownies

Prep Time: 15 Mins // Cook Time: 35 Mins

Thanksgiving | Christmas | New Year | Easter

Servings: 6

These are awesome! I have done this a few times and will continue to make them as the entire family love them... You can top these with coconut whip cream

Ingredients:

- 1/2 Cup Melted Coconut Oil
- 1/2 Cup Cocoa Powder
- 3/4 Cup Monk Fruit/Stevia Sweetener (Add more or less depending on sweet tooth)
- 2 Flax Eggs (1 Tbl Grounded Flax Seeds and 3 Tbl Spring Water becomes One Egg - You Need Two)
- 1/2 Tsp. Pink Salt
- 1 Tsp. Espresso or Whisky or Non Dairy Milk(Coconut milk)
- 1 Tsp. Vanilla
- 1/4 Cup Chocolate chips of Cacoa Nips
- 1/4 Cup Coconut Flour

Instructions:

1. Pre heat oven 350F, in a sauce pan, Combine the Coconut Oil, Cocoa Powder, Chocolate –
2. Medium heat, Whisking until mixture is smooth and No Lumps
3. Take off heat and stir in the sweetener
4. Add in the Flax eggs and Vanilla, mix well, add in the coconut flour, salt, espresso , mix well
5. Pour in pan and Bake for 15-20 Minutes, let cool completely then Serve.
6. Enjoy!

Chocolate Cake

Prep Time: 15 Mins // Cook Time: 35 Mins

Thanksgiving | Christmas | New Year | Easter | Birthday

Servings: 6

If you love chocolate cake, then you'll love this chocolate cake! It's nice and soft very moist - Not dry at all. This will MELT IN YOUR MOUTH!!!!!

Ingredients:

- 1/2 Cup Coconut Oil
- 1/4 Cup Monk Fruit/Stevia Sweetener (Add more if you like, depending on taste)
- 3 Eggs Room Temperature
- 1 Tsp. Vanilla Extract
- 1 1/2 Cup Almond Flour (As find as you can get it)
- 1/3 Cup Coconut Flour
- a Pinch of pink Himalayan Salt
- 2 Tsp. Baking Powder
- 1/4 Tsp. Xanthan gum
- 1/3 Cup Cocoa or Cacao Powder
- 1 Cup Vanilla Almond Milk or Unsweetened

Instructions:

1. Pre heat oven 350F
2. Grease pan with Coconut oil, blend all Ingredients in blender for a couple of minutes till nice and smooth
3. Bake for 50-60 minutes, let it cool for 10-15 minutes before cutting!
4. Enjoy!

Blueberry Muffins

Prep Time: 10 Mins // Cook Time: 30 Mins

Thanksgiving | Christmas | New Year | Easter | Halloween

Yield: 12

Serving Size: 1 Muffin

Ingredients

- 1/2 cup coconut flour
- 6 tablespoons psyllium husk
- 1 teaspoon baking powder
- 1/2 teaspoon salt
- 1/2 cup unsweetened sunflower seed butter
- 1/4 cup softened coconut oil, ghee or tallow
- 4 large eggs, room temperature
- 3 tablespoons yacon syrup or 1/3 cup honest syrup
- 1/2 cup non-dairy milk of choice
- 1 teaspoon vanilla extract
- 2 tsp. lemon zest
- 1 cup blueberries

Instructions

17. Preheat oven to 350F. Line a muffin tin with cupcake liners.
18. In a large bowl whisk together the coconut flour, psyllium husk, baking powder and salt.
19. In a separate bowl beat together the sunflower seed butter, coconut oil, eggs, syrup, vanilla and milk until well combined and creamy.
20. Add the wet mix to the dry mix and beat until a dough forms.
21. Add in the blueberries and lemon zest and use a spatula to fold in.
22. Use a ¼ cup scoop per muffin. Bake in the center rack for 25- 30 minutes or until the muffins have risen, round and golden on top.
23. Coconut Flour Blueberry Muffins (paleo, keto, dairy free, nut free)

24. Remove from the oven and let cool. Store in an airtight container at room temperature for up to 5 days.

Recipe Notes:

You can also use Zero Syrup which is vegetable glycerin (a sugar alcohol) and monk fruit or Honest Syrup made of vegetable fiber and monk fruit. While the latter is free of sugar alcohols which is ideal for some, it is high very high in total carbs (fiber). Use 1/4 to 1/3 cup in this recipe instead of Yacon Syrup.

Calories: 176.2, Fat: 12.7g, Carbohydrates: 10.4g, Fiber: 6.5g, Protein: 5.2g

Chocolate Hazelnut Spread Swirl Muffins

Prep Time: 10 Mins // Cook Time: 30 Mins

Thanksgiving | Christmas | New Year

Servings: 6

Calories: 255kcal

Make 6 muffins at 5 net carbs each.

These delicious Sugar-Free and low carb nutella swirl muffins feature a moist almond flour muffin base made in the blender. They're perfect for any ketogenic diet.

Ingredients

DRY INGREDIENTS

- 1 1/2 cups Almond Flour (130 g)
- 1 tbsp. whey protein isolate (optional)
- 1 tsp. baking powder
- 1/4 tsp. salt

WET INGREDIENTS

- 1/2 cup coconut heavy cream
- 2 large eggs
- 1 1/2 tsp. vanilla extract
- 1/3 cup Sukrin :1(Sugar-Free granulated sugar alternative)

SWIRL TOPPING

- 6 tsp. Sukrin Sugar-Free Chocolate Hazelnut Spread (homemade Nutella)

Instructions

PREPARATION:

1. Preheat oven to 350 degrees F and place rack to the middle position. Line 6 regular sized muffin wells with parchment liners.
2. Warm the Sukrin Chocolate Hazelnut Spread in the microwave for 20-30 seconds or until it is easy to drizzle from a teaspoon.

METHOD:

1. Put the wet ingredients into the blender.
2. Then put the dry ingredients into the blender. Turn the blender on low and blend. Remove the lid and help the process out with a spatula.
3. Turn up to medium low and blend for 20 seconds or until the batter is smooth and nicely aerated.
4. Divide the muffin batter between 6 muffin wells, filling 3/4 full. Drizzle 1 teaspoon of the Sukrin Chocolate Hazelnut Spread over each muffin and swirl/mix with a toothpick.

BAKE:

1. Bake for 25-35 minutes or until the tops of the muffins are firm and springy to the touch but still sound moist.
2. Let cool for 5 minutes in the muffin tin then remove to a cooling rack. Refrigerate in an airtight container for 7-10 days or keep on the counter for up to 5 days.

NOTES

The protein powder helps the muffins keep their shape and not collapse in the middle once the hazelnut spread is added. I did not use it in the muffins in the pictures and you can see a dip where they collapsed a bit. They are still delicious, but are better with the protein powder. I'll leave the choice up to you.

NUTRITION

Blackberry Custard Pie - Easy Coconut milk Pie Recipe

Prep Time 10 minutes // Cook Time 10 minutes

Thanksgiving | Christmas | New Year | Easter | Halloween

Servings 10

Calories 355kcal

Blackberry custard pie features an easy buttermilk custard pie filling in a pre-baked pie crust with fresh blackberries. This no-bake pie recipe cooks in minutes and is sugar-free.

Ingredients

- 1 recipe Basic Low Carb Pie Crust or your favorite 9-inch pie crust recipe)
- 1 cup Coconutmilk
- 3/4 cup coconut heavy cream
- 5 tbsp Tagatesse (or 1/2 cup Sukrin :1 or Swerve Granulated) (If not low carb use 1/2 cup sugar)
- 1/4 tsp xanthan gum
- 4 large eggs
- 2 large egg yolks
- 1 tsp gelatin powder (bloomed in 1 tbsp water)
- 1 tsp vanilla extract
- 1 pinch salt
- 1 pinch ground nutmeg

Instructions

Preparation

1. Sprinkle gelatin over 1 tablespoon water to bloom. Measure sweetener, salt and xanthan gum in a 4-6 cup capacity non-reactive metal pot.
2. Add the eggs and yolks and whisk together until completely combined. Whisk in the Coconutmilk and coconut heavy cream.

Cook

1. Place the pot over medium heat, whisking constantly until the mixture begins to thicken - about the 5 minute mark if using Tagatesse and 8 minutes for Sukrin :1 or Swerve.
2. Turn the heat down to medium low and whisk vigorously for 1 minute. (The custard should bubble lazily if whisking stops.) Remove from heat and whisk for 1 1/2 minutes more.
3. Tear the gelatin into pieces and drop into the custard, stirring until dissolved. Add vanilla and nutmeg, stirring to blend.

Assemble

1. Let the mixture cool just slightly then pour into pre-baked pie crust. Level the top and arrange black berries, pushing them into the custard until they are at least 1/2 way submerged.
2. Refrigerate uncovered for several hours before covering with cling film. Chill at least 6 hours before slicing and serving.

Optional Step

1. Sprinkle Tagatessse [Sukrin Melis, Swerve Confectioners] over the top and brown with a culinary torch.
2. Pay particular attention to the black berries to make them look like they baked.

Calories: 355kcal | Carbohydrates: 10g | Protein: 16g | Fat: 28g | Fiber: 4g

APPETIZER

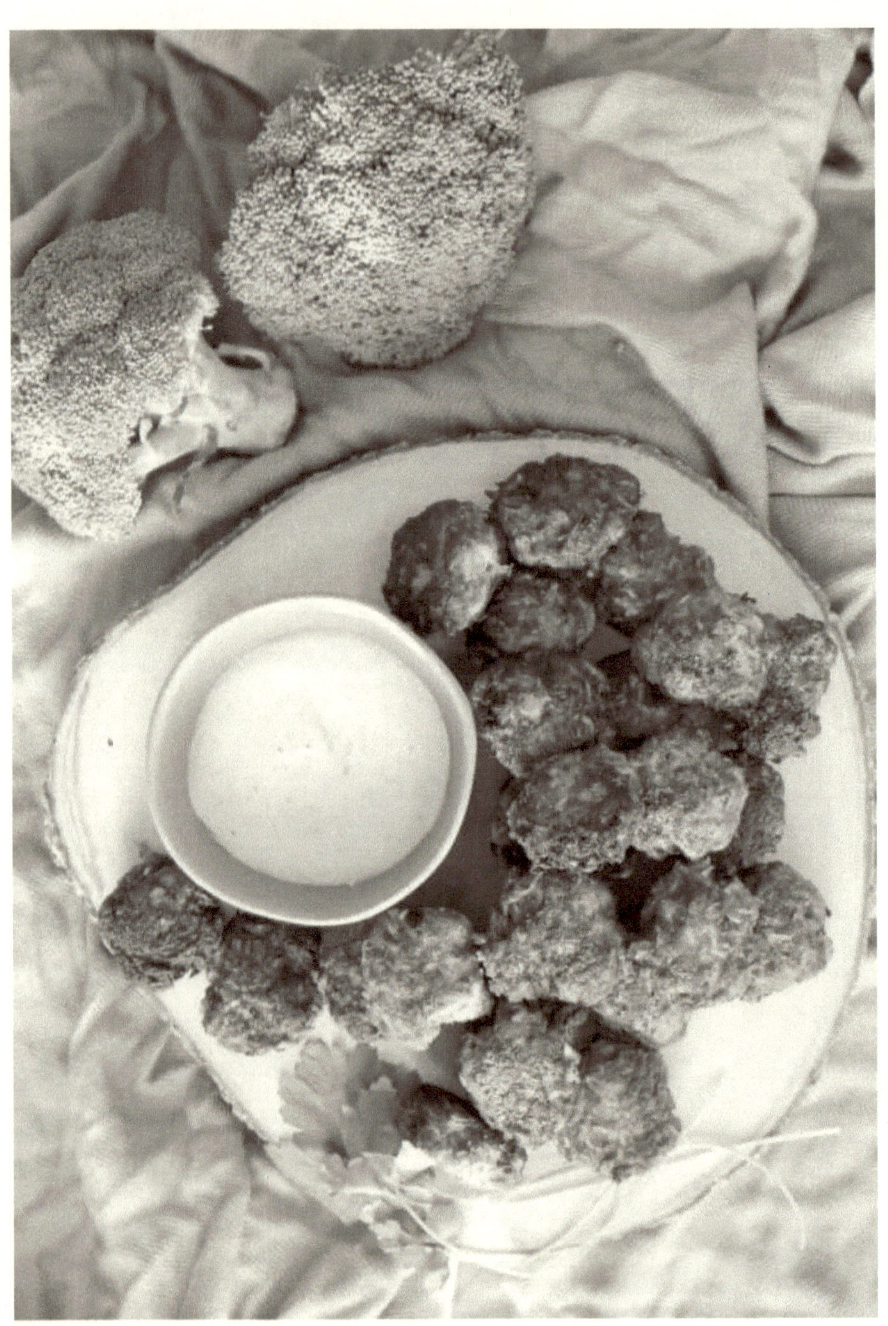

Keto Egg Roll Poppers

(Paleo, Flourless, Dairy Free)

Prep Time: 15mins // Cook Time: 30 mins

Thanksgiving | Christmas | New year| Birthday

Yield: 35 poppers

Category: appetizer or side

Serving Size: 5 Poppers Dipped In Sauce

We've all seen, heard of or tried a keto egg roll on a bowl recipe. I mean, they're taking over the internet. Shredded veggies, usually a blend of something cruciferous, sautéed with ground pork or turkey. Seasoned with delicious takeout flavors like sesame or soy.

Yeah, it's a great, one skillet meal. Delicious and easy keto egg roll poppers! Ground pork, broccoli and Asian seasonings in a delicious fried finger food!

Ingredients

- 1/4 cup coconut oil (for frying)
- 4 cups shredded broccoli (I use leftover stalks for this)
- 2 pounds ground pork
- 4 cloves garlic, fine minced
- 2 tablespoons fresh minced ginger, mince so fine it's like a paste (or 2 teaspoons ground ginger)
- 3 teaspoons fine salt
- 2 teaspoons ground mustard seeds
- 1 teaspoon black pepper
- 3 teaspoons coconut aminos
- 3 ounces pork panko (ground up pork rinds)
- 2 large eggs

For The Sauce:

- 1/3 cup coconut yogurt (see post for substitutions)
- 1 tablespoon sesame oil
- 1 tablespoon sesame seeds (or everything bagel seasoning)
- 1 teaspoon fresh ginger
- 1 tablespoon coconut aminos
- splash of fish sauce

Instructions

1. Heat your broccoli slaw in a large skillet with a tight-fitting lid with 2 tablespoons water for 10 minutes over medium heat.
2. Let it cool then strain it through a fine-mesh sieve, kitchen towel or nut milk bag, you want to remove as much water as possible. Alternatively, you may microwave the slaw for 2 minutes on high heat before straining the water out.
3. Heat a large skillet over medium heat with the coconut oil while you prepare the mix and the poppers.
4. In a large bowl combine the pork, broccoli, garlic, ginger, salt, black pepper, mustard seed, coconut aminos, pork panko and eggs.
5. Mix well until evenly combined. Shape 35 small balls and gently flatten. Check the oil, when a wooden spoon inserted sizzles, it's ready to fry.
6. Fry 6-7 poppers in the hot coconut oil, 3 minutes per side. Don't overcrowd the skillet. I use a 9″ cast iron skillet for this.
7. If your skillet is larger you will need add extra oil so it's high enough to pan fry. It should come up to half way up the poppers when 6-7 are in the oil.
8. Fry in batches until all the poppers are done. As you remove from the oil, place them on a paper towel lined plate.

Make the sauce: combine all of the sauce ingredients in a bowl and stir well.

Recipe Notes:

You can use a MICROPLANE to get the garlic and ginger in a fine mince for this recipe, easier than using a knife!

Calories: 485, Fat: 36g, Carbohydrates: 7g, Fiber: 3g, Protein: 33g

Bacon Wrapped Steak Bites

Prep Tim: 5 mins // Cook Time: 15 mins

Thanksgiving | Christmas | New Year

Servings: 8

Calories: 168 kcal

Thesebacon wrapped steak bites are easy to make and perfect for entertaining. Everyone loves bacon and steak and they tend to disappear quickly.

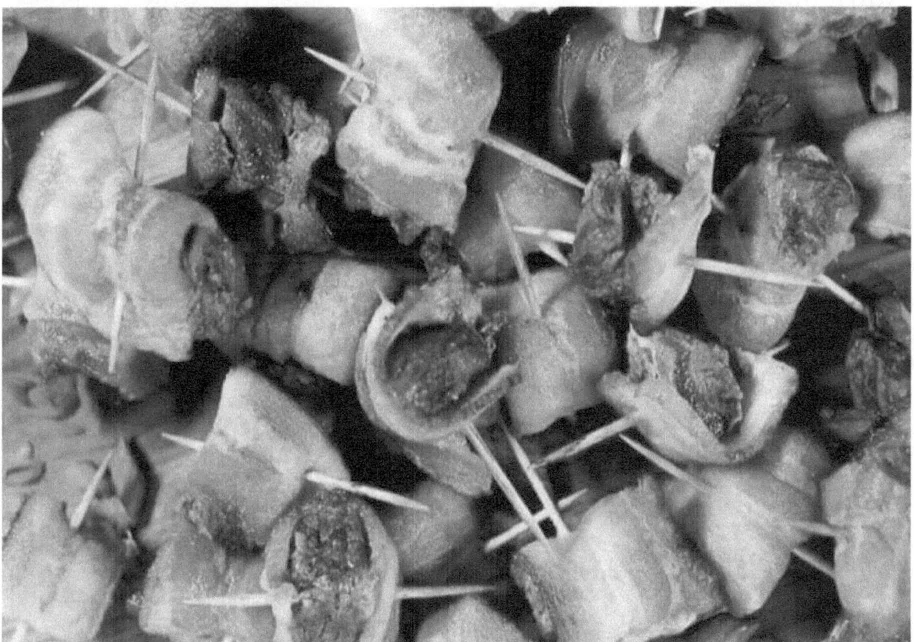

Ingredients

- 1 pound grass fed beef or elk (Sirloin, beef tenderloin medallions, elk backstrap, etc. Anything that can be cut into bite-sized pieces for cooking)
- 8 pieces of bacon
- Salt & pepper

Instructions

1. Preheat the oven to 425° Fahrenheit.
2. Cut your beef into small, bite-sized cubes. You want them bite-sized and a big mouthful can be tough to chew.

3   Season the beef cubes with salt and pepper.
4   Cut each strip of bacon into thirds.
5   Wrap the bacon around the beef cubes and secure it with a
    toothpick. Place on a baking tray.
6   Bake the bites in the oven for about 12-15 minutes, until the bacon
    starts to get crispy and the steak is cooked. If needed, you can switch
    the oven to broil at the end to crisp up the bacon.
7   Serve and enjoy.

Recipe Notes

Nutrition facts are an estimate provided for those following a
Ketogenic or low-carb diet. See our full nutrition information
disclosure here. The serving size for this recipe is 3 steak bites.

**Calories 168 Calories from Fat 99, Fat 11g17%, Protein
15g30%**

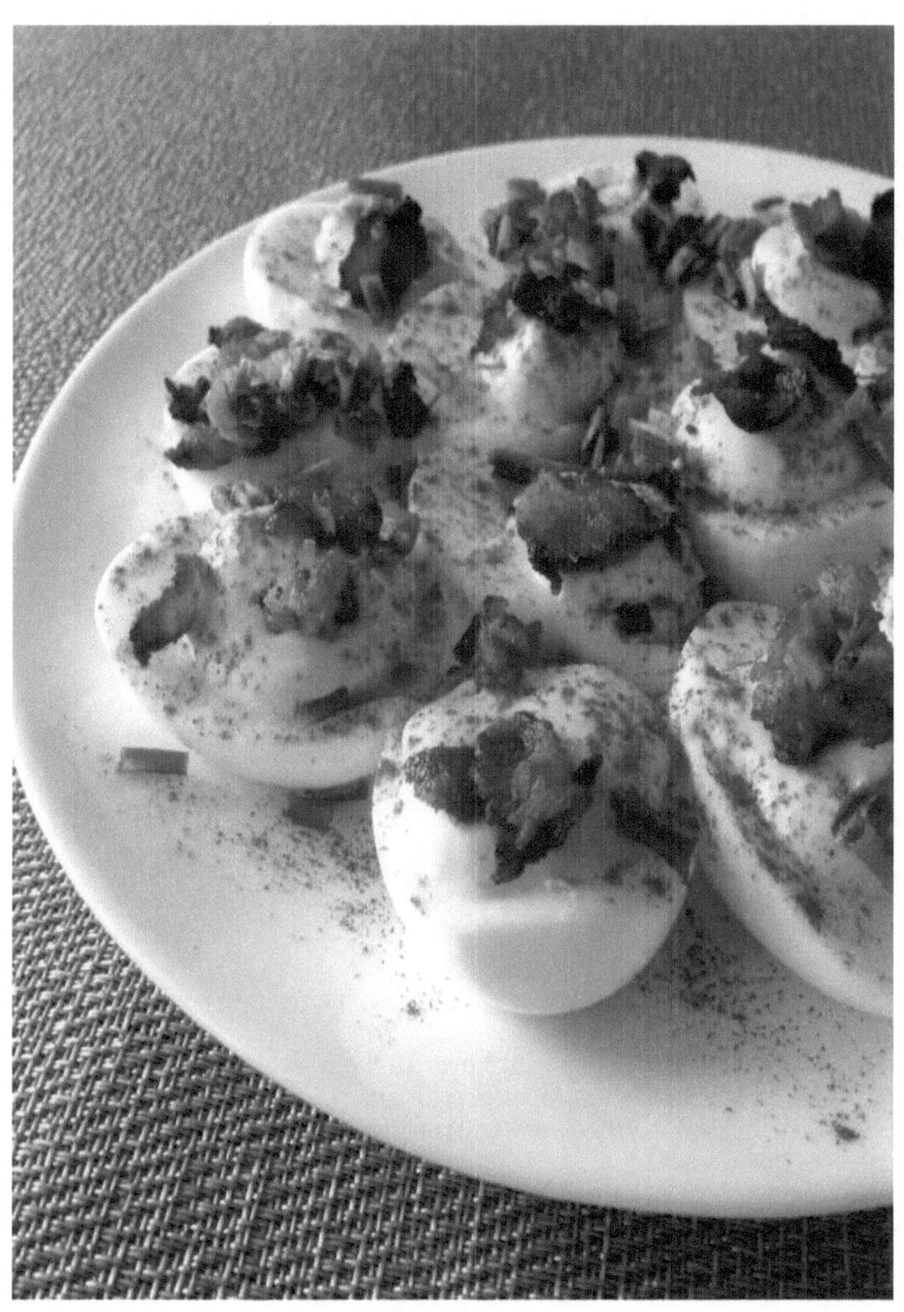

Bacon Deviled Eggs

Prep Time: 30 minutes//Cook Time: 5 minutes

Thanksgiving | Christmas | New Year

Servings: 6 servings

A paleo and low FODMAP version of deviled eggs, made with homemade mayonnaise, and topped with crispy bacon and fresh chives.

Ingredients

- 6 eggs hard boiled
- 1/2 cup homemade mayo - see link to my recipe above - or preferred mayo
- 1 tbsp + 1 tsp brown or dijon mustard
- 1/4 tsp fine grain sea salt
- 2-3 slices nitrate free bacon
- 2 tbsp thinly sliced fresh chives or green onions
- 1/2 tsp smoked paprika

Instructions

1. Peel your hard boiled eggs and cut each one in half lengthwise. Carefully remove the yolks and put them in a medium bowl. Set the egg white halves aside for the meantime.
2. Cook the bacon over med-hi heat in a heavy skillet until crisp, then drain, crumble, and set aside.
3. Mash the hardboiled egg yolks with a fork, then add the mayo, mustard, and salt and mix very well, until you have a thick, creamy filling for the whites. Alternatively, you could beat with a hand mixer to get a smooth consistency.
4. Carefully spoon the yolk mixture into the egg white halves, about 1-2 tbsp per half or enough to overfill a little.
5. Sprinkle the smoked paprika over all the eggs, then top with the crumbled bacon and chives or scallions.
6. Serve right away, or cover tightly with plastic wrap and store in the fridge until serving.
7. Enjoy!

Rosemary Roasted Turkey

Prep Time: 5 minutes//Cook Time: 35 minutes

Thanksgiving | Christmas | New Year | Easter | Halloween

Course: Appetizer, Snack

Servings: 8 servings

A holiday feast wouldn't be complete without a golden roasted turkey. Rosemary is our first choice when enhancing the flavor of poultry, and it fills the home with a wonderful aroma during cooking. This recipe is one to enjoy with your entire family or loved ones for any holiday.

Ingredients

- 2 Tbsp Extra Virgin Olive Oil
- 2 Tbsp fresh Rosemary, roughly chopped
- 7 lb Turkey Breast
- 2 tsp Salt and Pepper, to taste

Instructions

1. Preheat oven to 325°F.
2. Drizzle olive oil over turkey breast, brush to coat.
3. Separate rosemary from stems, roughly chop and sprinkle liberally on turkey.
4. Add salt and cracked pepper to taste.
5. Place turkey in shallow roasting pan.
6. Cook turkey approximately 25 minutes per pound (turkey is done when a meat thermometer inserted into the breast reads 170°F).
7. Periodically baste turkey with juices in the pan, especially toward the end of the cooking.
8. Let rest for 10 minutes, carve, and serve.

Spicy Baked Shrimp with Cilantro Lime Dip

Prep time: 5 Mins // Cook time: 10 Mins

Thanksgiving | Christmas | New Year | Easter | Halloween

Serving Size: 1 /yield: 4

Calories 481

For punch in the face flavor, make these Cilantro Lime Spicy Baked Shrimp! This Whole compliant recipe starts with shrimp covered in spices, baked to perfection then served with a fresh cilantro lime dip. Perfect for a healthy lunch, dinner, appetizer or a snack!

Ingredients

Spicy Shrimp

- 1 Lb . Large Wild Shrimp - thawed, peeled, deveined, tail-on
- 2 Tablespoons Olive Oil, (or avocado oil)
- 1/2 teaspoon Chili Powder
- 1/2 teaspoon Garlic Powder
- 1/4 teaspoon Cumin
- 1/4 teaspoon Onion Powder
- 1/4 teaspoon Sea Salt, or Kosher
- 1/8 teaspoon Ground Pepper

Cilantro Lime Dip

- Juice of 2 Small Limes
- Zest of 1 Lime
- 1/4 Cup Olive Oil, (or avocado oil)
- Handful Fresh Cilantro - stems removed, chopped
- Pinch Sea Salt

Instructions

1. Preheat oven to 400°F
2. Rinse and Drain thawed shrimp.
3. Toss shrimp with oil and spices. Transfer to a rimmed baking sheet.
4. Bake 8-10 minutes (depending on size) or until shrimp are pink and in a loose 'C' shape.

Cilantro Lime Dip

- Whisk all ingredients for 1-2 minutes.

- Serve with shrimp.

Serving Size: 1

Amount Per Serving

Calories 481, Total Fat 33,g Saturated Fat 5g, Trans Fat 0g, Unsaturated Fat 26g, Cholesterol 239mg, Sodium 1299mg, Carbohydrates 22g, Fiber 7g, Sugar 8g, Protein 28g

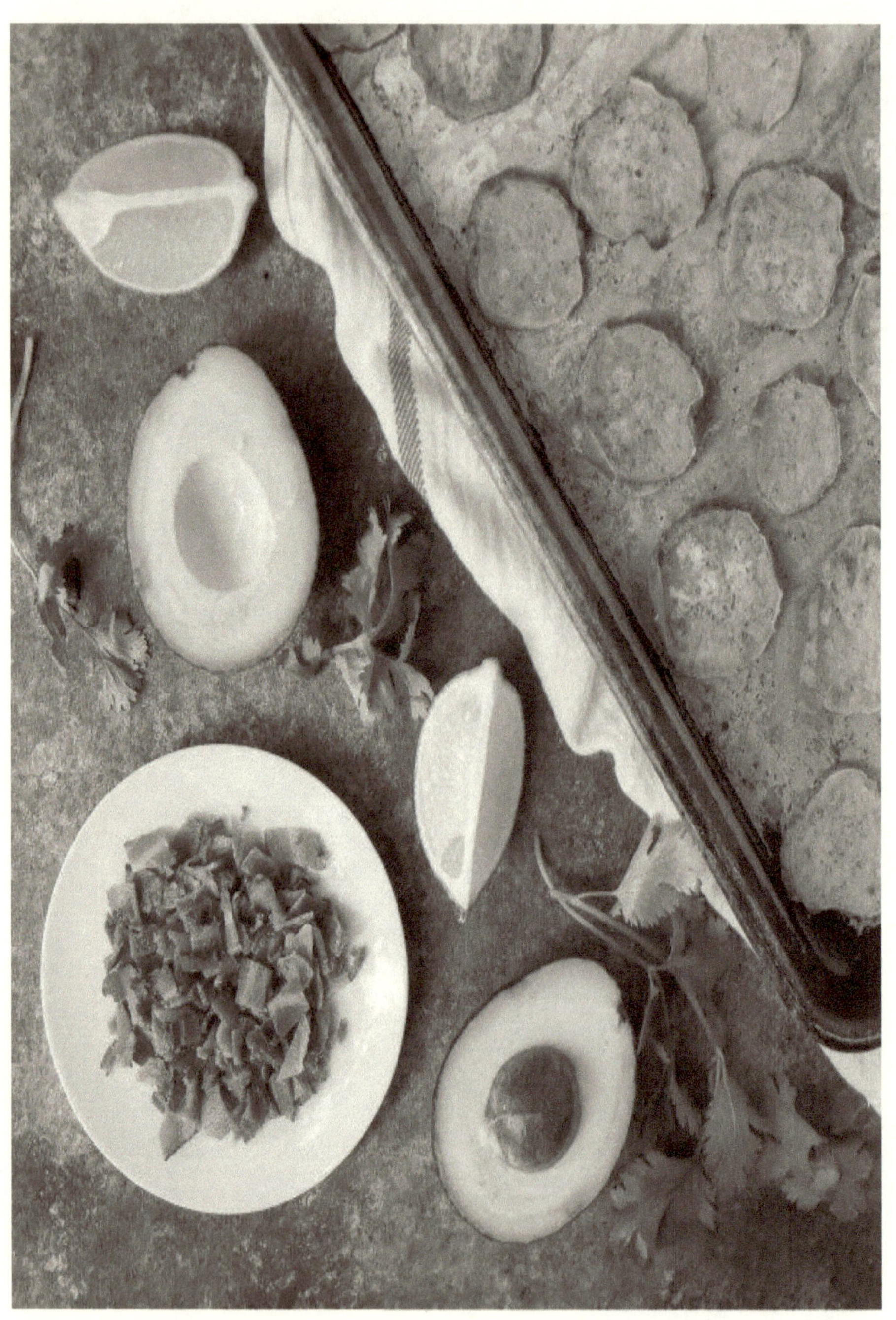

Sweet Potato Bites with Avocado and Bacon

Prep time:15 Mins // Cook time:30 Mins

Thanksgiving | Christmas | New Year | Easter | Halloween

Yield: 40 Bites

Course: Appetizer

Baked Sweet Potato Bites topped with avocado, bacon, and cilantro. This easy, crowd-pleasing appetizer is always a hit at parties! Gluten free and Paleo.

Ingredients

- 4 slices thick-cut bacon — about 3 ounces
- 2 tablespoons extra-virgin olive oil
- 2 sweet potatoes — scrubbed clean, peels on
- 1 1/4 teaspoons kosher salt — divided
- 3/4 teaspoon black pepper
- 2 medium avocados — peeled, pitted, and diced
- 1 tablespoon fresh lime juice
- 1/2 teaspoon smoked paprika
- 3 tablespoons chopped cilantro

Instructions

1. Preheat oven to 400 degrees F. Bake bacon according to these directions. Remove to a paper towel–lined plate and lightly pat dry. Once cool enough to handle, dice and set aside.
2. If necessary, move the racks to the upper and lower thirds of the oven. Increase the oven temperature to 425 degrees F. Line two rimmed baking sheets with foil (if reusing one of the bacon sheets, change out the foil for a fresh piece).
3. Brush sheets with 1/2 tablespoon olive oil each. With a mandoline or very sharp knife, slice the sweet potatoes into 1/2- to 1/4-inch slices.
4. Arrange the slices in a single layer on the oiled baking sheets, then brush tops with the remaining 1 tablespoon olive oil.
5. Sprinkle with 1 teaspoon salt and black pepper. Bake for 20 to 25 minutes, until golden brown underneath, rotating the pans 180 degrees and changing their positions on the upper/lower racks halfway through. Remove the pans from the oven, flip the slices over, then roast for an additional 8 to 11 minutes, until golden on top.

6   Meanwhile, in a small bowl, combine the avocado, lime juice, remaining 1/4 teaspoon salt, and smoked paprika. Mash lightly with a fork, leaving the mixture slightly chunky. Set aside.

7   Transfer the baked sweet potato slices to a serving plate. Top each with a dollop of the avocado mixture, chopped bacon, and cilantro. Serve warm or at room temperature.

Recipe Notes

Make ahead tips:

- Slice the sweet potatoes and bake the bacon up to 1 day in advance. Store separately in airtight containers in the refrigerator.
- The avocado mixture can be made a few hours in advance. Store in the refrigerator with plastic wrap pressed tightly against the top to prevent browning.
- I recommend baking the sweet potatoes and assembling the bites as close to serving time as possible, as they do become a bit soggy as they sit.
- Even if they do soften somewhat, they will still be delicious!

Amount per serving (1 bite) — Calories: 31, Fat: 2g, Cholesterol: 1mg, Sodium: 52mg, Carbohydrates: 3g, Fiber: 1g, Sugar: 1g, Protein: 1g

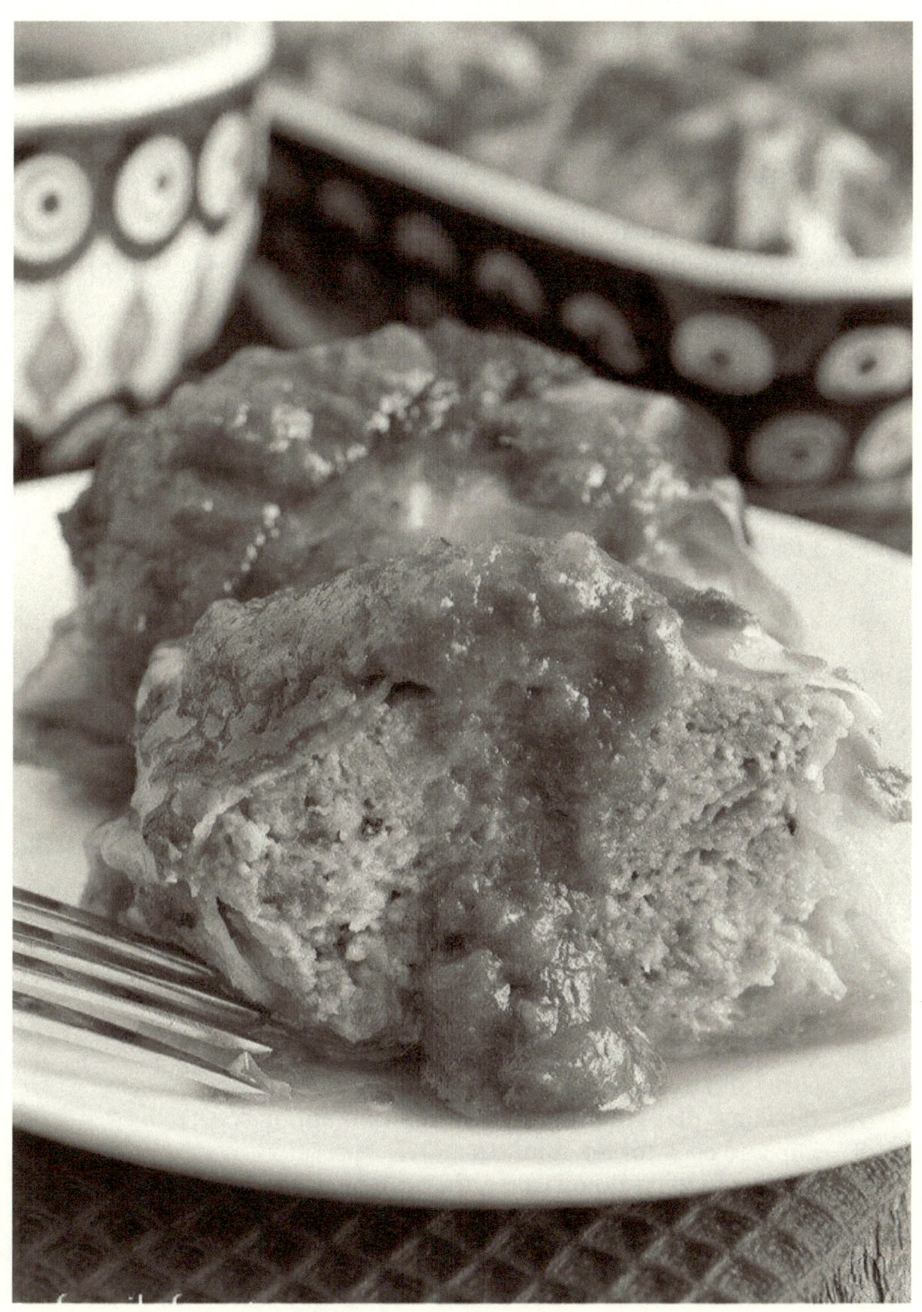

Whole Salmon Cakes

Prep Time: 15 mins // Cook Time: 30 mins

Thanksgiving | Christmas | New Year

Yield: 7 cakes

Ingredients

- 1 14.75-ounce can wild-caught salmon
- 1 cup cooked sweet potato (canned with no syrup is OK to use)
- 1 whole egg
- ½ cup almond flour
- 2 tablespoons minced fresh parsley
- 2 scallions sliced thin, tops and bottoms, roots removed
- 2 teaspoons dried dill
- 1 teaspoon hot sauce (optional)
- ½ teaspoon paprika
- 1 teaspoon kosher salt
- ¼ teaspoon freshly ground black pepper
- 2 tablespoons clarified coconut oil, melted

Instructions

Note: These can be made ahead and frozen and baked frozen if desired.

1. If baking immediately, preheat oven to 425 degrees F.
2. Line a small sheet tray with parchment paper.
3. Drain liquid from can of salmon and discard liquid. Pick out bones and skin and discard. Take remaining salmon, break into pieces and place in a medium bowl.
4. Add all other ingredients except coconut oil.
5. Mix and form into seven equal patties about 1" thick.
6. Oil parchment paper and set salmon cakes on paper. If freezing, cover and freeze.
7. If baking, place in preheated oven for 20 minutes.
8. Flip and cook for ten minutes more.
9. If using frozen salmon cakes, they can be baked frozen or thawed. If baking frozen, you may need to adjust cooking time.
10. Serve with tartar sauce (see recipe below) and lemon.

Whole Tartar Sauce

Prep Time: 15 mins // Total Time: 15 mins

Thanksgiving | Christmas | New Year

Yield: 1 cup

Ingredients

- ½ cup Olive Oil Mayonnaise
- 1 Tablespoon minced cornichons or dill pickle
- 2 Tablespoons minced fresh flat leaf parsley
- 2 teaspoons minced capers
- 2 teaspoons minced fresh chives
- ½ tablespoon fresh lemon juice
- 1 teaspoon pickle juice
- Salt to taste
- Freshly ground black pepper to taste

Instructions

1. Place all ingredients in a bowl and mix to combine. Refrigerate for 30 minutes before serving.

Paleo Coconut Shrimp Recipe

Prep Time: 10 Minutes Cook Time: 25 Minutes

Servings: 6

Ingredients

- cups 100% pineapple juice
- 1/4 cup coconut palm sugar
- 1 pound jumbo shrimp peeled and veined
- 1/2 cup unsweetened shredded coconut flakes
- 1/4 cup almond flour
- 1 teaspoon sea salt
- 1/8 teaspoon garlic powder
- 1/8 teaspoon ground cayenne pepper

Instructions

2. Preheat the oven to 400 degrees F. Line a couple baking sheets with parchment paper and set aside.
3. Pour the pineapple juice in a small sauce pot and add the coconut sugar. Bring to a boil. Once boiling, lower the heat and simmer for 10-15 minutes to allow the juice to reduce to 1/2 cup liquid. Once it forms a thick syrup, remove from heat and pour in a shallow dish to cool.
4. Pour the shredded coconut, almond flour, salt, garlic powder, and cayenne in a bowl. Stir to combine.
5. Pat the shrimp dry with a paper towel. When the pineapple syrup has cooled and is just barely warm, toss the shrimp into the syrup to thoroughly coat.
6. Dip each shrimp into the coconut mixture to cover with crust, then lay them out on the baking sheets. Bake for 8-10 minutes until the shrimp is cooked through and the crust is slightly golden. Serve warm!

Calories: 212kcal, carbohydrates: 19g, protein: 17g, fat: 8g, saturated fat: 4g, cholesterol: 191mg, sodium: 992mg, potassium: 201mg, fiber: 2g, sugar: 13g, vitamin a: 15iu, vitamin c: 11mg, calcium: 131mg, iron: 2.3mg

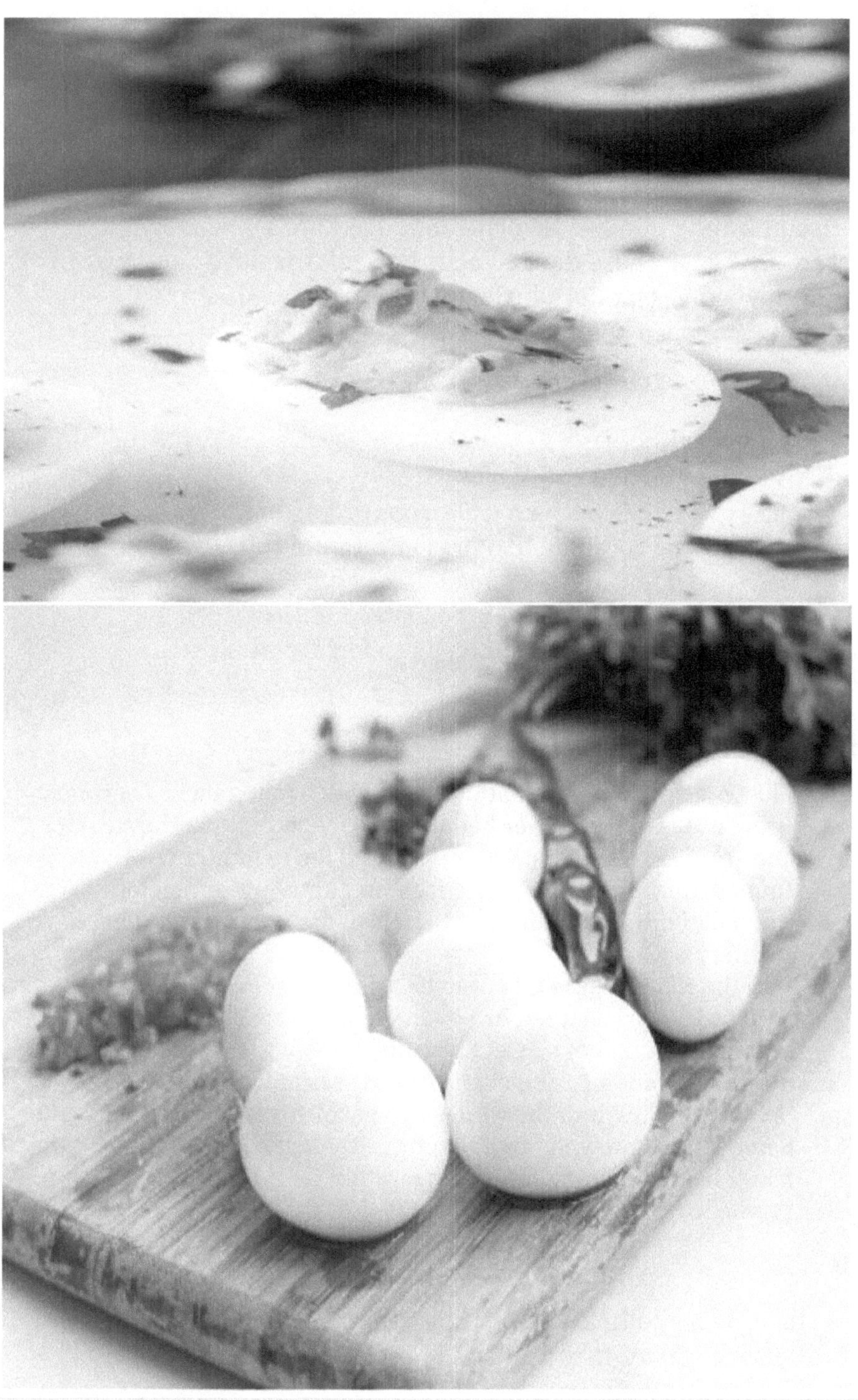

Deviled Guacamole Eggs

Prep Time: 10 Minutes Cook Time: 25 Minutes

Thanksgiving | Christmas | New Year | Easter | Halloween

Serves Makes 16 (halves)

We're combining our two favorite appetizers into one: Deviled Guacamole Eggs! These deviled eggs have all the flavor and pizazz of regular deviled eggs, plus a little guacamole kick. They are mayonnaise free, so healthy to boot!

Ingredients

- 8 eggs
- 1/2 large avocado
- juice of 1/2 lime (about a tablespoon)
- 1 tablespoon coconut oil, room temperature
- dash of hot sauce
- 1/2 roma tomato or 3 cherry tomatoes, minced
- 1 tablespoon cilantro, minced, plus more for garnish
- salt and pepper to taste

Instructions

1. Fill a pot with a steamer attachment with about 3 inches of water. Bring water to a boil over high heat. Place the eggs in the steamer and set over the boiling water with a lid for 12 minutes.
2. Immediately plunge eggs into ice water and cool completely. (You can boil them for 12 minutes directly in the water if you don't have a steamer.)
3. Peel the cooled eggs and cut in half. Put the yolks into the bowl of a food processor, blender, or bowl. Add the avocado, lime juice, coconut oil, and hot sauce. Pulse until smooth, or mash with a fork.
4. Stir in the tomatoes and cilantro, and season with salt and pepper.
5. Spoon the filing into the whites and garnish with extra cilantro. Serve immediately. If you are serving them later, store them in the fridge but let come to room temperature for 30 minutes before serving.

Notes

These have avocado in them, so they will brown if you wait a while before serving. Cover them tightly.

Bacon Wrapped Shrimp

Prep Time: 5 Minutes // Cook Time: 6 Minutes

Thanksgiving | Christmas | New Year | Easter

yield: 16

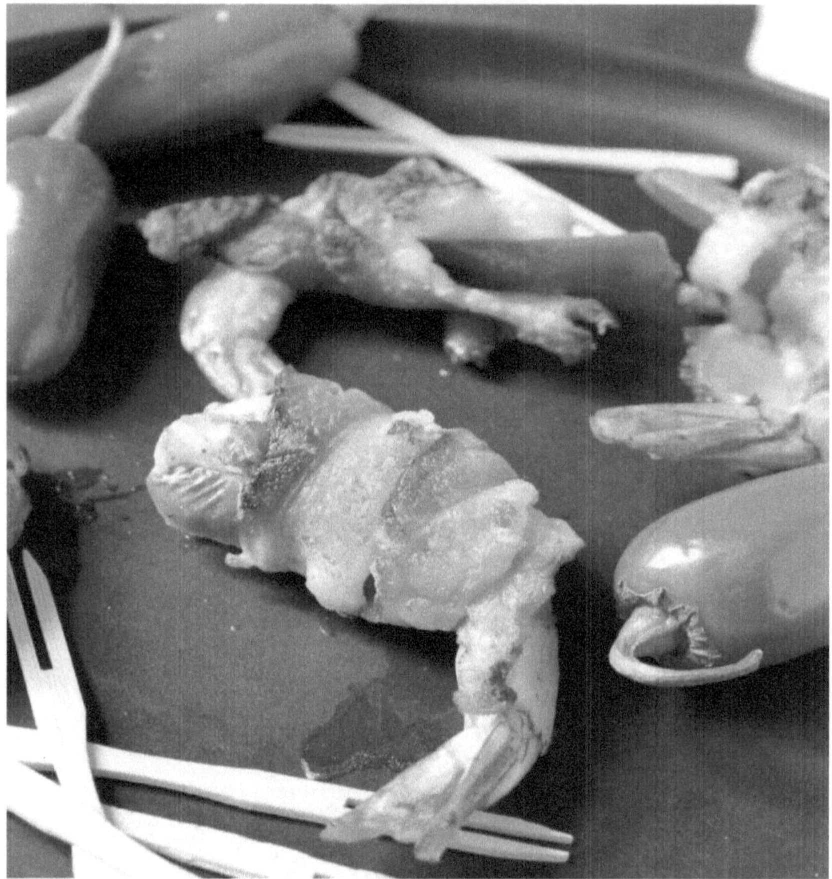

These Bacon Wrapped Shrimp are a quick and simple appetizer, perfect for holidays, game day or parties. Just wrap shrimp and jalapeño with bacon and fry it up. These can also be made Whole - Paleo compliant.

Ingredients

- 16 extra-large shrimp, peeled, deveined, and tails removed (about 12 ounces)
- 1 jalapeño chile, stem removed, seeded, and cut lengthwise into 16 thin strips

- 1 teaspoon kosher salt
- 1 teaspoon black pepper
- 8 bacon slices, halved lengthwise

Instructions

1. Heat a skillet or grill pan over medium. Cut a long 1/4-inch-deep slit in the inner curve of each shrimp; insert 1 jalapeño strip.
2. Sprinkle with the salt and pepper. Wrap each shrimp tightly with 1 bacon piece. Set on a plate, seam sides down.
3. Place the bacon-wrapped shrimp, seam sides down, in the hot skillet, and cook, turning occasionally, until the bacon is crisp and the shrimp are just cooked through, 5 to 6 minutes.

Sausage and Cranberry Stuffed Mushrooms with Sage

Prep Time: 15 Minutes // Cook Time: 25 Minutes

Thanksgiving | Christmas | New Year

Servings: 30 Mushrooms

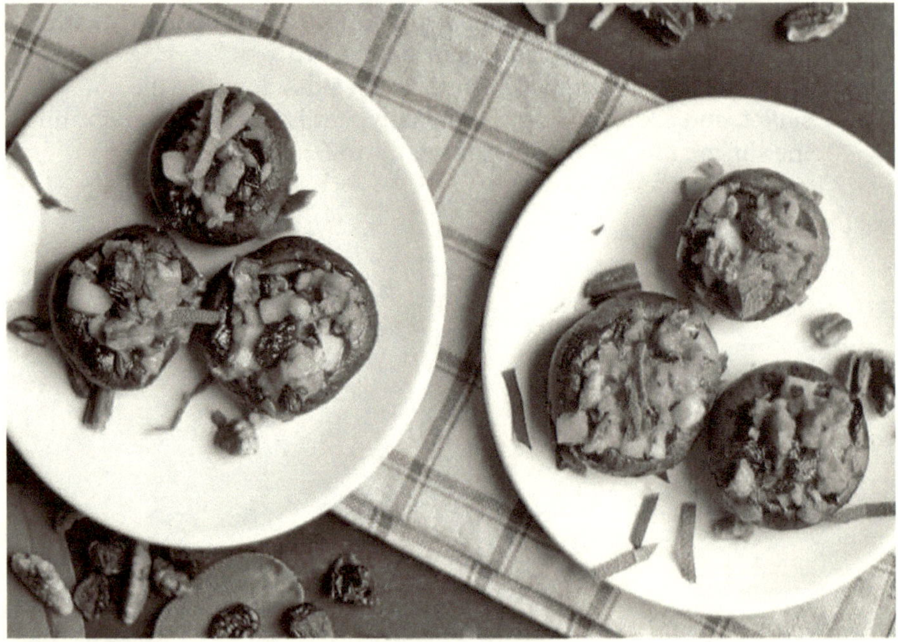

Ingredients

- 8 oz ground sausage
- 30-35 large white button or baby bella mushrooms stems removed
- 1/2 cup skinned cored, and chopped apples (really tiny pieces, or even shredded)
- 1/4 cup chopped leeks
- 1/4 cup finely chopped pecans
- 3 tbsp olive oil or avocado oil divided
- 1/3 cup chopped dried cranberries
- 2 tbsp chopped fresh sage
- 2 eggs beaten
- 1 clove garlic minced

Instructions

1. Preheat your oven to 350 degrees. Lightly grease a large baking sheet, set aside.
2. Heat up a large skillet to medium high heat. Coat with 2 tbsp oil, add sausage and begin to cook. Cook for about 2-3 minutes, add in leeks, apples, and pecans. Saute for another 4-5 minutes, or until sausage is cooked completely. Continue to break apart the sausage so there are no big chunks.
3. Pour mixture into a medium sized bowl. Add in cranberries, fresh sage, and eggs. Stir around so all ingredients are well mixed.
4. Mix the remaining oil with crushed garlic. Place the mushrooms inside the baking sheet, and brush the caps of each mushroom with oil/garlic mixture.
5. Spoon the mixture in each mushroom cap.
6. Place inside the oven and bake for 25 minutes, or until mushrooms are browned. Serve hot!

MAIN DISH

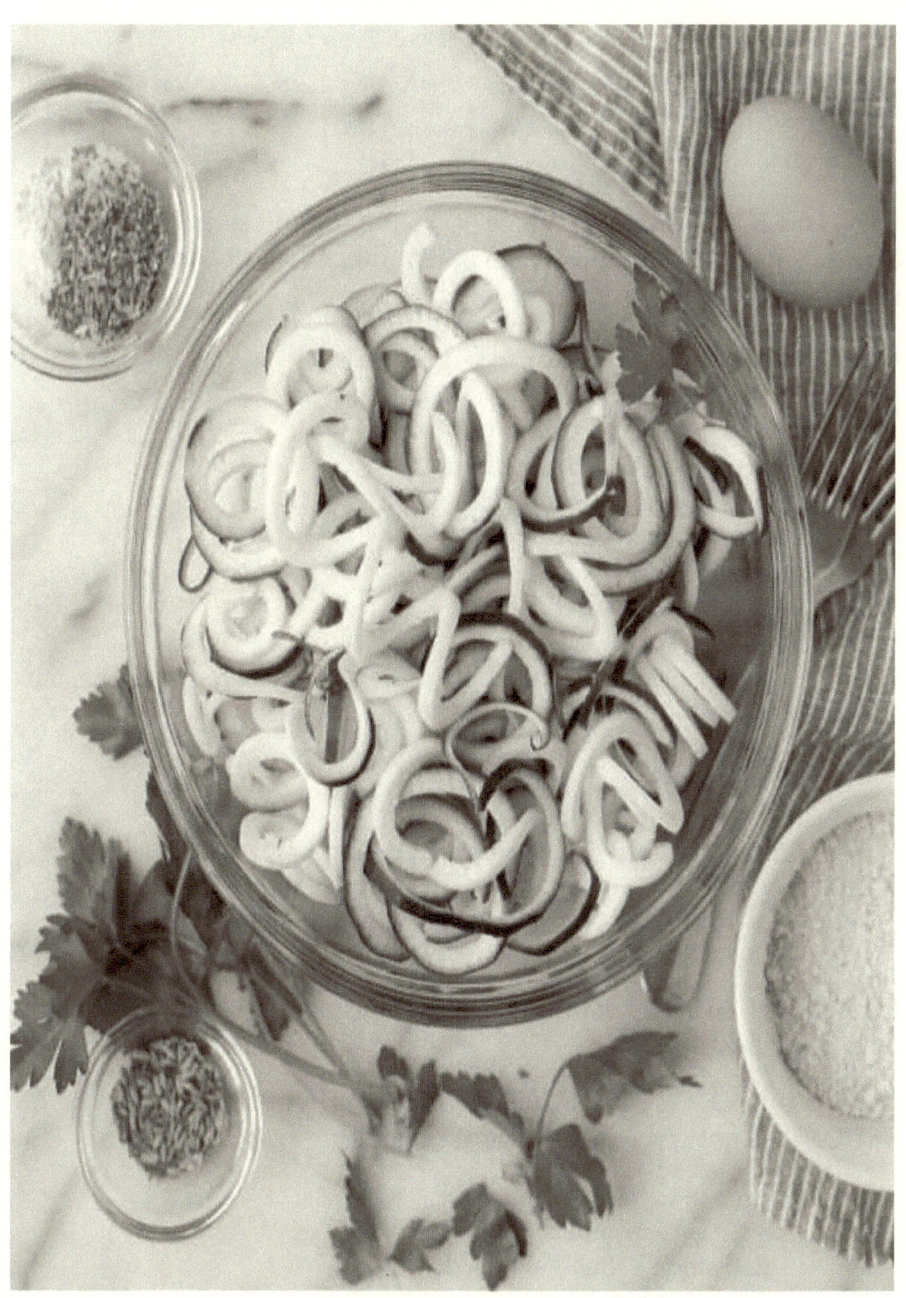

Meatballs and Sauce

Prep Time:25 mins||Cook Time:15 mins

Thanksgiving | Christmas | New Year | Easter | Halloween

Yield: 34 meatballs

Course: Main Course

Easy, DELICIOUS Italian Whole 30 meatballs and sauce with ground turkey, almond flour, and Italian seasoning. A healthy, low-carb recipe that families love!

Ingredients

FOR THE MEATBALLS:

- 1/4 cup blanched almond flour
- 1 1/2 teaspoons garlic powder
- 1 1/2 teaspoons dried oregano
- 1 teaspoon onion powder
- 1 teaspoon fennel seeds
- 1 teaspoon kosher salt
- 1/2 teaspoon crushed red pepper flakes — reduce to 1/4 teaspoon if sensitive to spice
- 1/4 teaspoon ground nutmeg
- 2 pounds 93% lean ground turkey
- 1 large egg — lightly beaten
- tablespoons finely chopped fresh parsley — plus additional for serving
- 24 ounces jarred prepared tomato-based pasta sauce* — or homemade pasta sauce, see below

For serving: Zucchini noodles — shredded spaghetti squash, or sweet potato noodles

IF YOU'D LIKE TO MAKE HOMEMADE WHOLE 30 MARINARA SAUCE (see notes for store-bought options):

- 1 teaspoon extra-virgin olive oil
- 2 cloves garlic — minced
- 1 small onion — finely chopped
- 1/2 teaspoon kosher salt
- 1/4 teaspoon black pepper
- 1 can crushed tomatoes — (28 ounces)

- 1 can diced tomatoes (I like to use fire roasted for extra flavor) — (14 ounces)
- 1 teaspoon dried basil
- 1/2 teaspoon dried oregano

Instructions

9. Place two oven racks in the upper and lower thirds of the oven. Preheat the oven to 400 degrees F.
10. Line two baking sheets with aluminum foil and lightly coat them with nonstick spray, or line them with parchment paper or silicone baking mats. (If you are making vegetable noodles to serve with the meatballs, I recommend prepping them now so that they are ready to serve when the meatballs finish cooking.
11. If you are making homemade sauce, I like to start this simmering before the meatballs go in the oven so that it is ready as well.)
12. In a small bowl, whisk together the almond flour, garlic, oregano, onion powder, fennel, salt, red pepper flakes, and nutmeg until the ingredients are evenly combined.
13. Add the turkey to a large bowl. Sprinkle the almond flour mix over the top. Add the beaten egg and parsley. With a fork or your hands, gently combine the ingredients until everything is evenly distributed.
14. Be careful not to overwork or compact the meat, or the meatballs will be tough.
15. With a small scoop or spoon, scoop the meat and shape into 1 1/2-inch balls, again being careful not to compact the meat. Arrange on the baking sheets. You will have about 34 meatballs total. If using store-bought sauce, warm it up while the meatballs cook.
16. Bake for 10 minutes, and then remove the baking sheet from the oven. Using tongs, gently turn the meatballs and return them to the oven, switching the position of the sheet pans on the upper and lower racks. Continue baking until cooked through, about 5 additional minutes. Serve hot with vegetable noodles, sauce, and a sprinkle of fresh parsley.

For Homemade Whole 30 Tomato Pasta Sauce:

4. Heat the olive oil in a large, deep skillet over medium high. Add the garlic, onion, salt, and pepper.
5. Cook for 5 minutes, until the onion is soft. Add the crushed tomatoes, diced tomatoes, basil, and oregano. Bring to a simmer.
6. Cook over medium heat until the sauce thickens slightly, stirring occasionally, about 14 minutes. Taste and adjust the seasoning with more salt and pepper as desired.

Recipe Notes

- *If purchasing pasta sauce, to keep the recipe Whole 30 compliant, ensure there are no added sugars or dairy in your sauce.
- Suggested brands I found online include Rao's Homemade Marinara Sauce, Mario Batali Tomato Basil Pasta Sauce, most Thrive Market sauces (aside from the vodka sauce, which has cream), and Trader Joe's Roasted Garlic Spaghetti Sauce (this is what I used).
- Be sure to double check the list of ingredients. You can also make the basic homemade spaghetti sauce I suggest above.

To freeze: Freeze with or without sauce for up to 2 months. Let thaw overnight in the refrigerator, and then reheat on the stove (with sauce to keep them from drying out).

Amount per serving (4 meatballs) — Calories: 185, Fat: 10g, Saturated Fat: 3g, Cholesterol: 23mg, Sodium: 236mg, Carbohydrates: 3g, Fiber: 1g, Protein: 26g

Turkey Burger with Crispy Kale (Keto, Whole, Paleo)

Prep Time: 15 Mins // Cook Time: 30 Mins

Thanksgiving | Christmas | New year| Birthday

Serving Size: 5

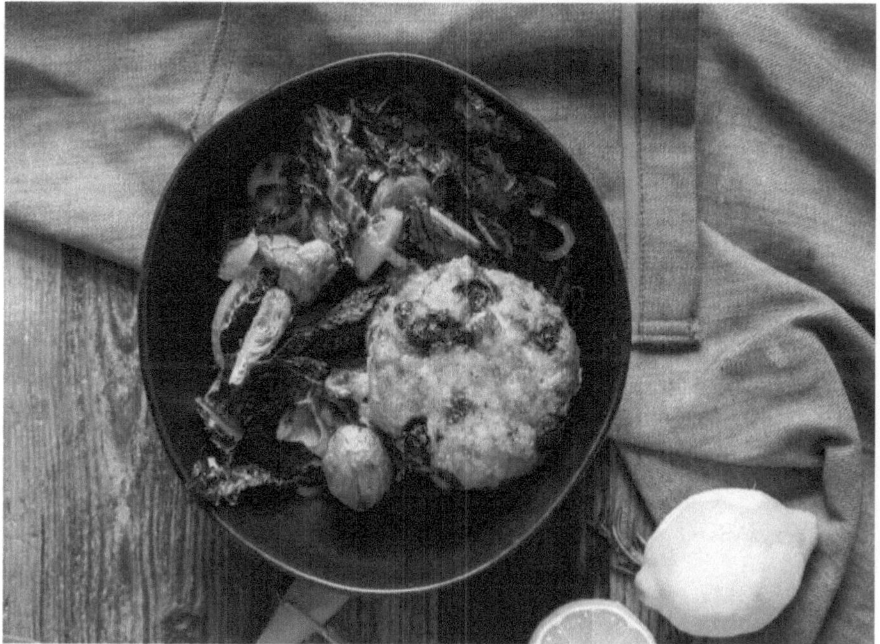

Ingredients

FOR THE TURKEY BURGERS

- 2 pounds ground turkey, dark meat
- 1 lemon, grated zest
- 2 sprigs rosemary needles
- ¼ cup fresh blueberries
- 2 teaspoon fine salt
- 2 tablespoons bacon fat, lard or ghee
- 1 large egg or 1 flax egg

FOR THE VEGETABLES

- 1 bunch dino kale, chopped
- 1 pound brussles, quartered
- ½ onion sliced

- 2 tbsp avo
- ½ teaspoon fine salt
- 1/2 teaspoon garlic powder
- 1/2 teaspoon ground pepper

Instructions

1. Pre-heat the oven to 400F. Make sure you have on rack in the center and one on the bottom.
2. In a large bowl combine all of the turkey burger ingredients. Mix well and shape 5-6 large turkey burgers. Place on an oiled sheet pan and set in the oven, middle rack. Set timer for 30 minutes.
3. Wash hands. On the second sheet pan combine all of the sliced and diced vegetables. Toss with avocado oil and seasonings using hands to massage the oil into the veggies.
4. Spread them out evenly over the sheet pan then place in the oven, bottom rack.
5. When the timer goes off. Remove everything from the oven!
6. Serve hot. Store leftovers in tupperware in the fridge for up to 5 days.

Pressure Cooker White Turkey Chili

Whole, Paleo

Prep Time: 10 mins//Cook Time: 30 mins

Thanksgiving | Christmas

Yield: 5

Category: Soup

Method: Pressure Cooker

A creamy, white soup with ground turkey, bacon and loads of flavor!

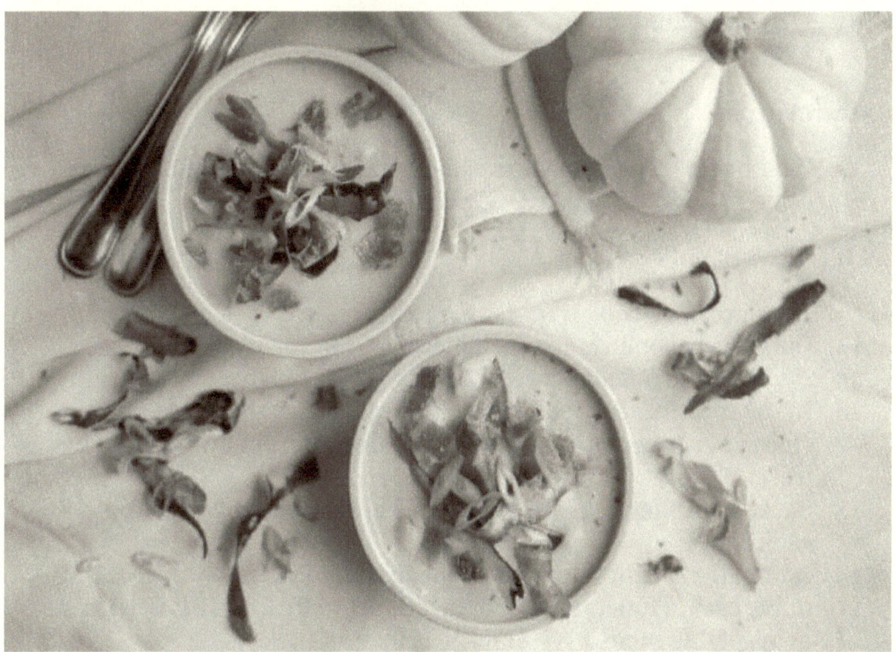

Ingredients

For Soup Base:

- 2 cups chopped leek whites
- 4–5 cups diced white sweet potatoes or 6 cups diced cauliflower
- 2 tbsp. bacon fat
- 1 tsp salt
- 1 tsp white pepper
- Pinch nutmeg
- 3 cups bone broth, more to taste
- 1 cup cashew or coconut cream

For Turkey

- 1–2lbs ground turkey
- ½ tsp salt
- ½ tsp mustard
- ½ tsp ground garlic
- ¼ cup minced leek greens
- 4 slices bacon

For Crispy Potato Skins *

- Sweet Potato Peels
- 1/4 cup coconut oil
- Skillet

Instructions

12. First begin by peeling your sweet potatoes and setting the skins aside, DO NOT DISCARD. Or dice your cauliflower.

START THE SOUP

13. Heat pressure cooker on saute mode.
14. Cut your bacon into 1/4 inch pieces.
15. Add it to the pot and cook until crispy.
16. In the meantime; slice your leeks until you hit the green part.
17. Once your bacon is crispy remove it from the pot and add in the leeks.
18. Saute until they begin to brown. Add in the sweet potato (or cauliflower)
19. Add in the broth, salt, white pepper and nutmeg.
20. Cancel saute function. Close the lid. Set to PRESSURE COOK: steam or vegetable mode.
21. During this time mix your ground turkey in a bowl with salt, mustard, ground garlic. Set aside.
22. Wash and mince the leek greens. Set aside.

MAKE CRISPY SKINS (IF USING POTATO)

6. Heat coconut oil in the skillet.
7. Line a plate with paper towel and set it close to the stove.
8. When a wooden spoon inserted in the oil sizzles, add in a handful of the potato skins.
9. Once they become golden brown (30-45 seconds) remove them with tongs and set on paper towel lined dish.
10. Repeat until all the skins are fried.

13. When the pressure cooker is done, release the pressure manually to speed up the process.
14. Then transfer all of the contents to a blender, carefully.
15. Place the insert back in the pot an heat on saute mode.
16. Add in the leek greens and ground turkey, saute until browned and cooked, about 5 minutes.
17. Stir often, you want to crumble the turkey with your spatula or spoon.
18. Blend the potato (or cauliflower) mix until smooth. Add in the cream. Blend again.
19. Pour your soup base into the pressure cooker and bring to a simmer with the turkey, this won't take but a minute or two.
20. If you want the soup thinner, add in more broth here. I like mine pretty thick!
21. Stir in MOST of the bacon, save some for garnish.
22. Serve soup. Top with crispy skins, bacon and green onion!
23. Boom! Delicious.
24. This will make a lot, about 5-6 bowls, which is about 8-10 cups.

Recipe Notes:

- AIP Modifications: Omit All The Seed Bases Spices Like Pepper, Nutmeg & Mustard.
- Use Horseradish, Ginger And A Little Cinnamon Instead.
- Use Coconut Cream Instead Of Cashew Cream.
- Ensure Your Bacon Is AIP Compliant.

Calories: 530, Fat: 34g, Carbohydrates: 17g, Fiber: 4g, Protein: 37g

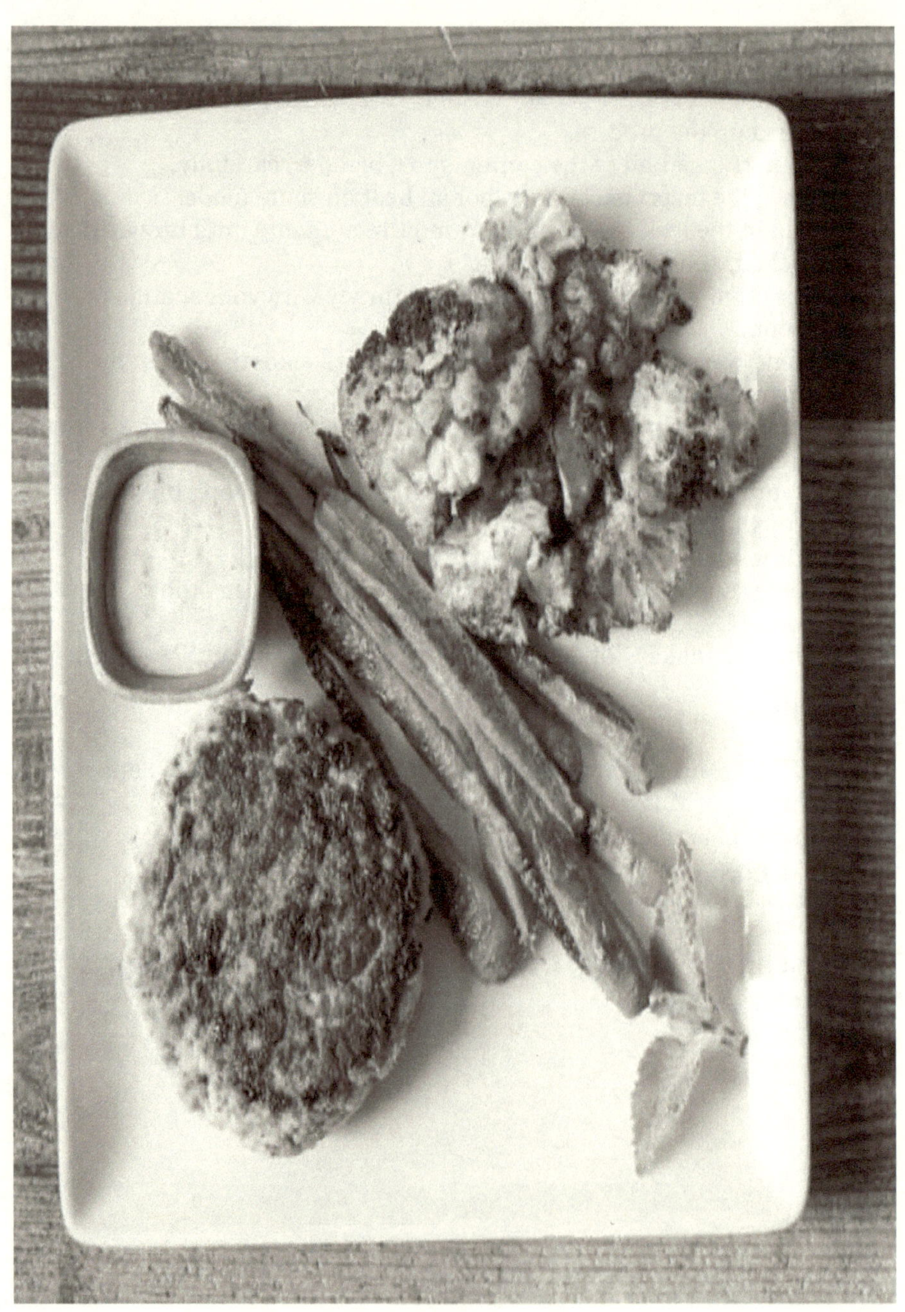

Strawberry Oregano Turkey Burgers

(Paleo, Nut Free)

Prep Time: 10 mins//Cook Time: 20 mins

Yield: 6

Thanksgiving | Christmas | Birthday

Serving Size: 1 Burger

Method: skillet

A surprisingly delicious combination!

Ingredients

- 2lbs ground turkey
- 1 strip cooked bacon (minced)
- 5 large strawberries (diced)
- 3 garlic cloves (minced)
- 2 tbsp fresh oregano (minced, you could use mint or basil too)
- 1.5 tsp salt
- 1 tsp pepper
- 1 egg
- 2 tbsp olive oil (more for cooking, could also use ghee)
- 1/2 cup coconut flour (sub fine ground almond meal)

Instructions

1. Prepare the strawberries, garlic, bacon, and oregano. Add to a large bowl.
2. Add in the turkey meat, egg, salt, pepper and olive oil. Mix well with a spatula or clean hands.
3. Pour coconut flour into a shallow bowl.
4. Heat a large cast iron skillet on medium heat until hot (sprinkle water, when it beads, it's hot). Drizzle in cooking fat.
5. Shape 6 large patties and gently toss them in the coconut flour. Use both hands to shape and handle until they feel more solid/dryer in your hands. If you're using almond meal just mix it into the meat.
6. Then add them to the skillet. I cook 2-3 at a time.
7. Brown 5 minutes on one side, then flip over. After 2 minutes, cover the skillet and cook another 3 minutes. Once they feel firm when you press down on the center, they are cooked through, or internal temp is 175F.
8. Repeat until all the patties are done.

Calories: 319, Fat: 17g, Carbohydrates: 10g, Fiber: 4g, Protein: 32g

Slow Cooker Turkey Breast - Paleo, Whole

Prep Time: 5 Minutes // Cook Time: 4 Hours 30 Minutes

Category: Main Course

Yield: 4

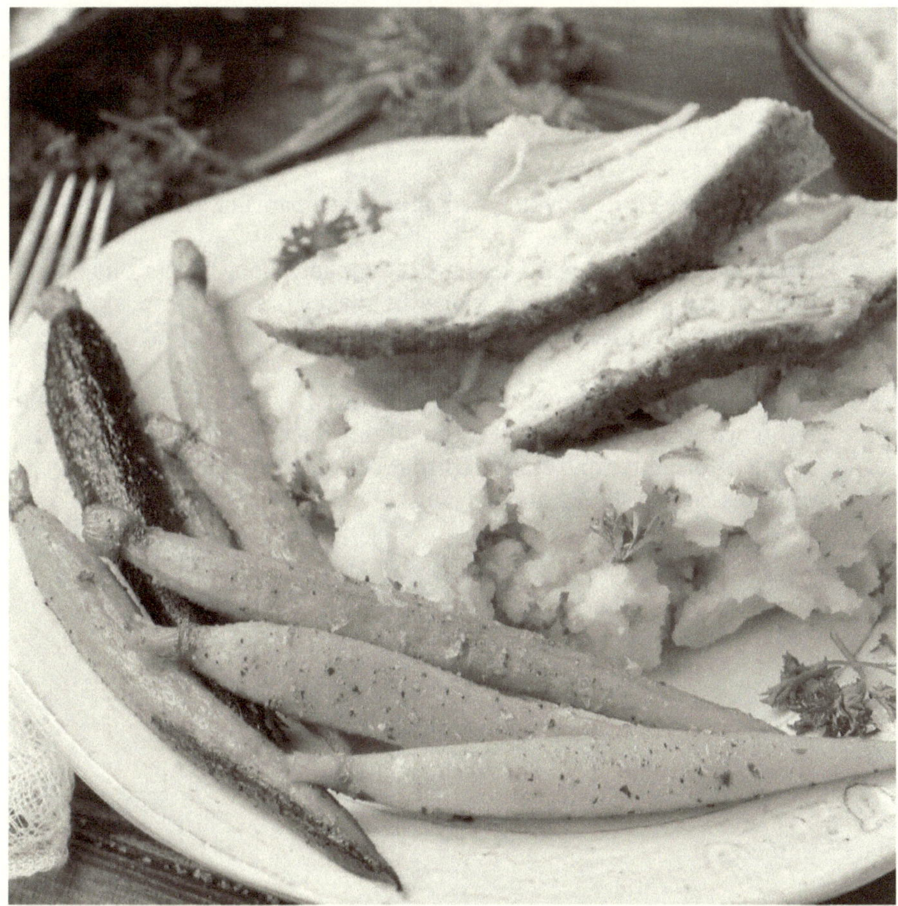

This Slow Cooker Turkey Breast is great for the holidays or as an easy dinner recipe year round! Add this to your small family holiday menu or make it as a nutritious meal. This is a Whole foods compliant and Paleo recipe.

Ingredients

- 1 teaspoon Garlic Powder
- 1 teaspoon Onion Powder

- 1/2 teaspoon Smoked Paprika
- 1/2 teaspoon Kosher Salt
- 1/2 teaspoon Ground Pepper
- Olive Oil
- 1 Sweet Onion, - cut into 1" rings
- 2 Lemons, - cut into 1/2" slices
- 3 Lb Halft Turkey Breast - skin on, bone in
- Fresh Rosemary
- Fresh Thyme
- Fresh Sage

Instructions

4. Mix together garlic powder, onion powder, paprika, salt and pepper. Set aside.
5. Drizzle olive oil inside a 6 quart slow cooker. Place the onions and lemons in a flat, even layer. Place the turkey breast on top, skin side up. Rub turkey breast with spices. Arrange fresh herbs around the turkey.
6. Cook on low for approximately 4½ hours. Begin checking internal temp every half hour at about the 3 hour mark. Once turkey reaches 165ºF internal temp, remove from crockpot. Allow to sit for 10-15 minutes before slicing and serving.

Thai Chicken Soup Recipe

Prep Time 5 minutes // Cook Time 20 minutes

Servings 4 -5

Thanksgiving | Christmas | Halloween

Calories 190 kcal

Course: Main Course

Paleo, Whole, Dairy Free, Gluten Free

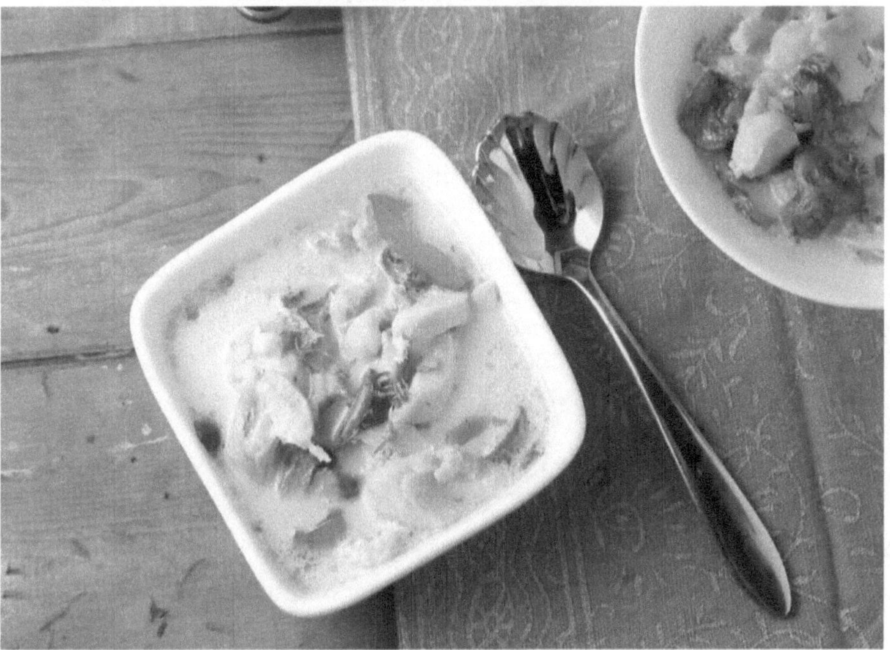

Ingredients

- 14 oz coconut milk this is my very favorite brand as it has no fillers/thickeners and amazing coconut cream!
- 2 cups chicken broth
- 6 slices FRESH ginger or galangal root about a quarter size each
- 1-2 lemongrass stalks cut into 3rds or 4ths, roughly smashed with a mallet or knife to release the flavor
- 1 pound boned and skinned chicken thighs cut into bite-size pieces
- cups sliced mushrooms I usually do a mix of cremini and shitake!
- 1 tablespoon lime juice or more taste
- 1 tablespoon fish sauce my favorite brand!!

- 1 teaspoon palm sugar or 4 drops liquid stevia, omit for Whole Foods
- 1-3 teaspoons Thai Chile Garlic Sauce or paste or sriracha, check label for added sweetener
- 1/2 cup fresh cilantro finely minced
- 1 teaspoon sea salt to taste

Optional:

- Lots of veggies would make a good addition to this soup..I love sweet peppers!

Instructions

5. In a soup pot, bring the coconut milk, chicken broth, ginger, and lemongrass to a boil.
6. Add the chicken and mushrooms and simmer until cooked through, about 10 minutes.
7. Remove lemongrass and ginger slices.
8. Add the remaining ingredients, more or less as you prefer!! Enjoy!

Calories 190 Calories from Fat 54, Fat 6g9%, Saturated Fat 2g13%, Cholesterol 107mg36%, Sodium 1471mg64%, Potassium 569mg16%, Carbohydrates 7g2%, Sugar 4g4%, Protein 24g48%, Vitamin A 160IU3%, Vitamin C 10.9mg13%, Calcium 59mg6%, Iron 1.5mg8%

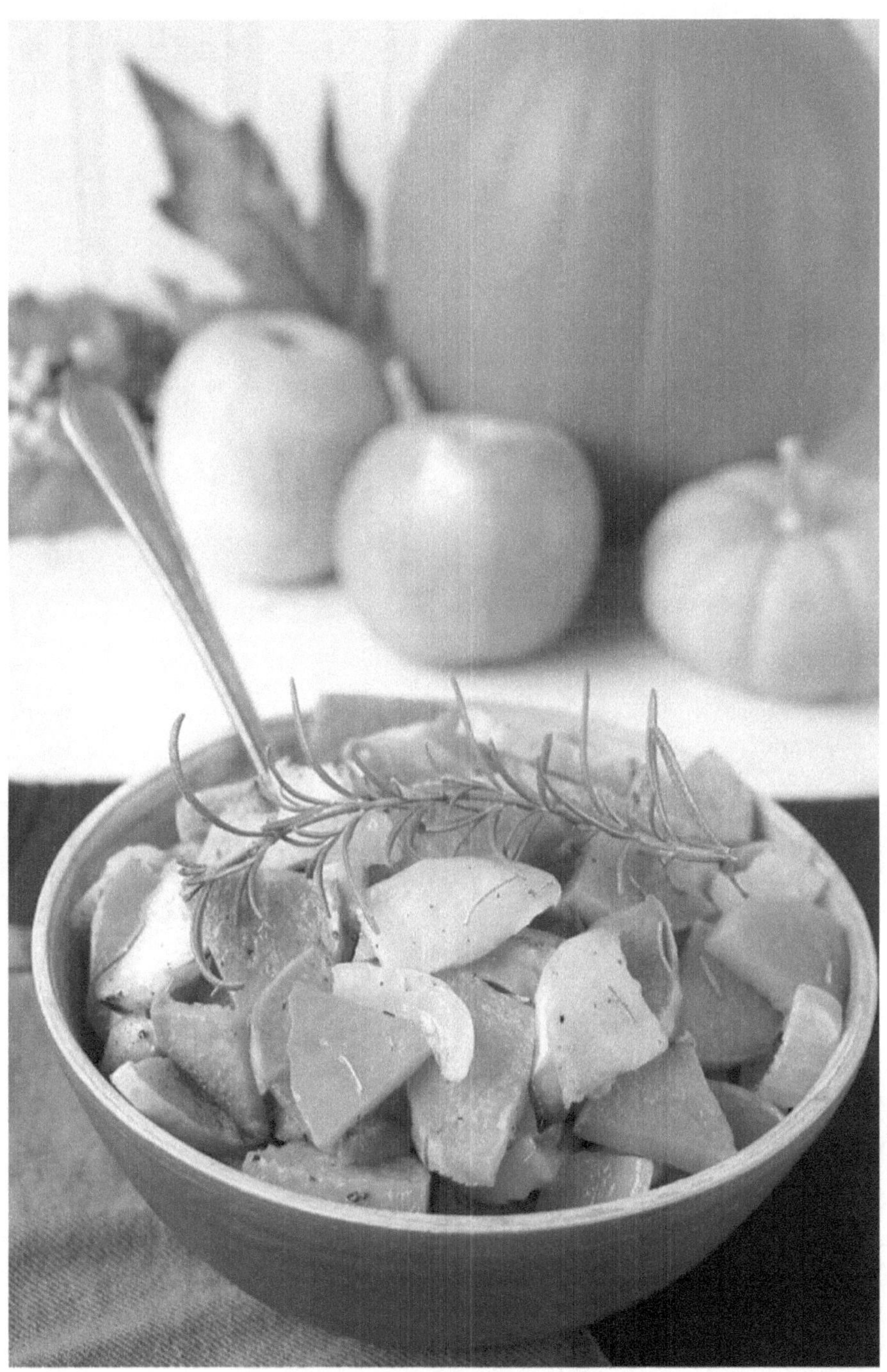

Roasted Sweet Potatoes, Squash, & Apples

Prep Time: 1 hr // Cook Time: 25 mins

Thanksgiving | Christmas | Halloween

Servings: 8 Servings

Course: Main dish

Ingredients

- 1 Extra Large Sweet Potato
- 1 Large Apple
- 1/2 Large Onion white or yellow
- 1 Honeynut Squash or 1/2 Butternut Squash
- Tbsp. Olive Oil
- 1 tsp. Dried Rosemary
- Salt and Pepper to taste

Instructions

6. Preheat oven to 400 degrees and line a baking sheet with parchment paper.
7. Chop sweet potatoes, squash, onion, and apple into bite-sized pieces and place on baking sheet.
8. Drizzle with olive oil and top with salt, pepper, and rosemary.
9. Bake for 20-25 minutes or until the vegetables are lightly browned on the edges.
10. Garnish with fresh rosemary

1-Dish Roasted Turkey Breast Dinner with Sweet Potatoes

Prep Time 10 minutes // Cook Time 2 hours 30 minutes

Thanksgiving | Christmas | New Year

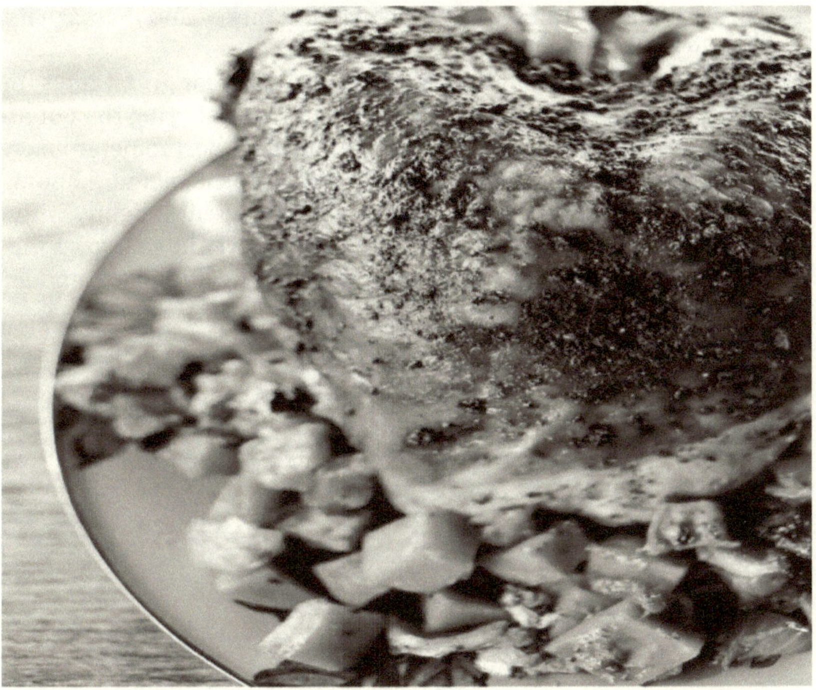

1-Pot Roasted Turkey Breast Dinner with Sweet Potatoes is so impressive, so delicious, and so easy that you'll make roasted turkey breast one of your regular meals!

Ingredients

- 2 large sweet potatoes peeled and cut into 1 1/2 to 2-inch cubes
- 2 large onions peeled and cut into 1 1/2 to 2-inch cubes
- 1 fresh or fully thawed frozen whole turkey breast 5 to 9 pounds
- 3 tablespoons canola or olive oil
- 1 apple cut into quarters
- the zest of one large orange
- 1 tablespoon of Cranberry Dry Rub per pound of turkey breast

Instructions

1   Preheat oven to 450°F. Scatter the sweet potato and onion chunks over the bottom of a small roasting pan or 9-inch by 13-inch, deep baking pan. Nestle the turkey breast into the sweet potatoes and onions. Drizzle the oil over the turkey breast and stuff the apple quarters into the turkey's cavity. Rub the orange zest all over the turkey breast.

2   Sprinkle the Cranberry Dry Rub over the turkey and massage it into the turkey breast with your hands.

3   Place the roasting pan into the oven and roast for 30 minutes, then lower the heat to 375°F and continue to roast, stirring the potatoes every 20 minutes or so, until an instant read thermometer inserted into the thickest part of the breast reaches 165°F, about 2 hours.

4   If the breast is browning too quickly, you can tent it lightly with foil.

5   When the turkey breast reaches 165°F, remove the pan from the oven, lay foil over the breast without crimping it in place, and let it rest for 10 minutes before carving.

Herbed Mayonnaise Roast Turkey

Prep time: 30 minutes // Cook time: 3 hours 30 minutes

Yield: 10 Pound Turkey

Thanksgiving | Christmas | New Year

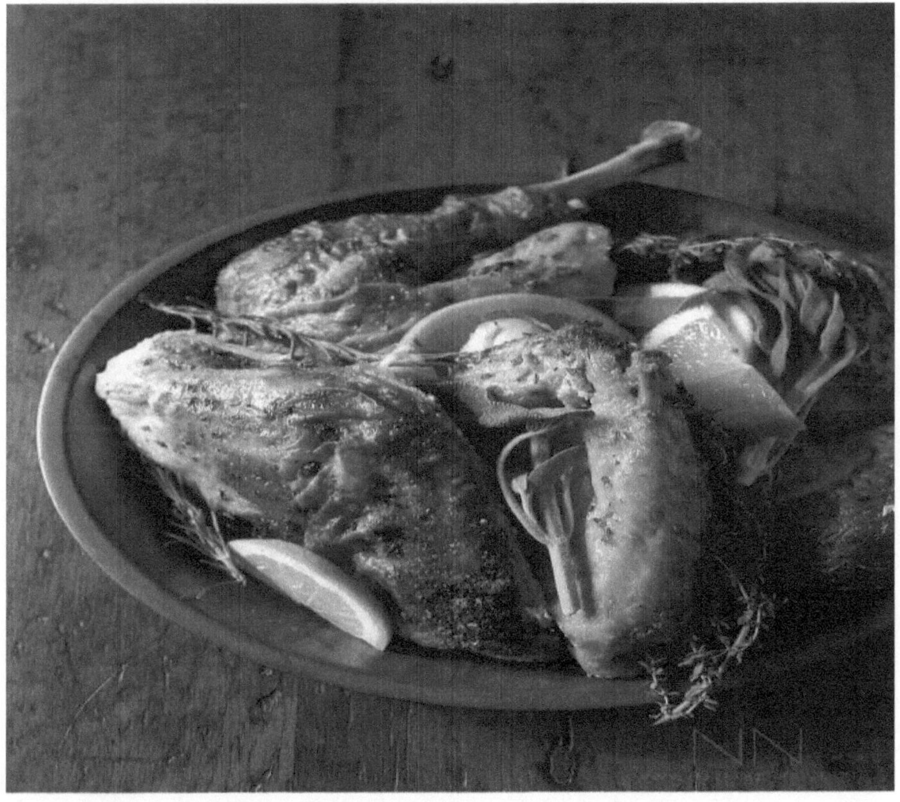

This herbed mayonnaise roast turkey is the perfect addition to your Thanksgiving table. Full of orange, sage, rosemary and thyme it's super moist and totally easy!

Ingredients:

- 1 (10 pound) fresh turkey (if using frozen make sure it's thawed)
- 1 cup mayonnaise
- 2 tablespoons orange zest
- 1 tablespoon minced fresh rosemary
- 1 tablespoon minced fresh thyme
- 1 tablespoon minced fresh sage
- 1 tablespoon orange juice

- Kosher salt and pepper, to taste
- 2 oranges, cut into wedges

Instructions

1. Preheat oven to 400 degrees.
2. Remove giblets from the inside of the turkey and add turkey to your roasting pan.
3. Using a paper towel lightly dry off the turkey skin.
4. In a small bowl whisk together mayonnaise, orange zest, rosemary, thyme, sage and orange juice.
5. Rub mayonnaise mixture over the entire turkey and inside the cavity. I use my hands for this job because it the easiest way to coat the entire turkey.
6. Sprinkle the turkey with kosher salt and pepper.
7. Stuff the cavity with orange wedges and any remaining fresh herbs you might have.
8. If you're using a popup timer simply place it into the meaty part of the breast. Press down into the turkey until the timer is flush with the skin.
9. Add turkey to the oven and cook for 30 minutes at 400 degrees. Lower temperature to 350 and cook until timer pops up or internal temperature is 180 degrees.
10. If the top of your turkey gets too browned while cooking simply tent it with foil for a bit then remove the foil to continue browning until fully cooked.
11. Let your turkey rest for at least 30 minutes (I usually let mine rest for about an hour) then carve and enjoy!

Orange Glazed Ham

Prep Time: 10 Mins // Cook Time: 1 Hour 30 Mins

Yield: 10 1x

Category: Main Entree

Thanksgiving | Christmas | New Year | Easter | Halloween

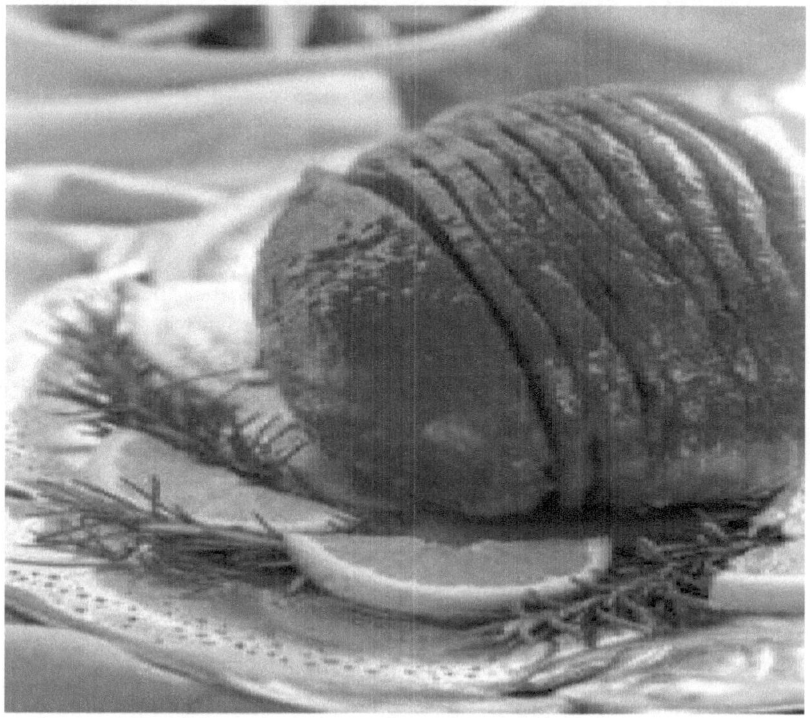

Now you can enjoy perfectly glazed ham without added sugar! Our baked ham with it's simple 4 ingredient orange and spice glaze is easy enough for a casual weekend dinner or meal prep session and elegant enough for holiday feasts.

Ingredients

- 4–5lb. Pederson's Natural Farms No-sugar Uncured Smoked Boneless Ham (or other fully-cooked ham)
- ½ cup water

For the Glaze:

- ¾ cup frozen orange juice concentrate, slightly thawed
- ⅓ cup water

- ¼ tsp. dried ground ginger (recommend Pure Indian Foods)
- ⅛ tsp. ground cloves

Instructions

1. Preheat oven to 325°F. Position oven rack in the lower ⅓ of the oven.
2. Unwrap ham and place sliced side down on a rack in roasting pan. Add ½ cup water to bottom of pan. Place a sheet of parchment paper over the ham then cover with aluminum foil.
3. Place pan in oven and roast 45 minutes.
4. While ham is in the oven, prepare glaze by adding orange juice, water, ginger and cloves to a small saucepan. Bring to a boil, reduce heat then simmer until reduced to roughly half and glaze is slightly thickened. Remove from heat.
5. After 45 minutes, remove ham from oven and uncover. Spoon or brush some of the glaze over ham. Return ham to oven uncovered.
6. Continue to spoon or brush remaining glaze over the ham every 15 minutes until a thermometer inserted in the center of the ham registers 140°F.
7. Remove ham from oven and allow to rest, covered, for 10 minutes before slicing and serving.

Prime Rib Roast Recipe

Prep Time: 15 Minutes // Cook Time: 3 Hours 30 Minutes

Thanksgiving | Christmas | New Year | Easter | Halloween

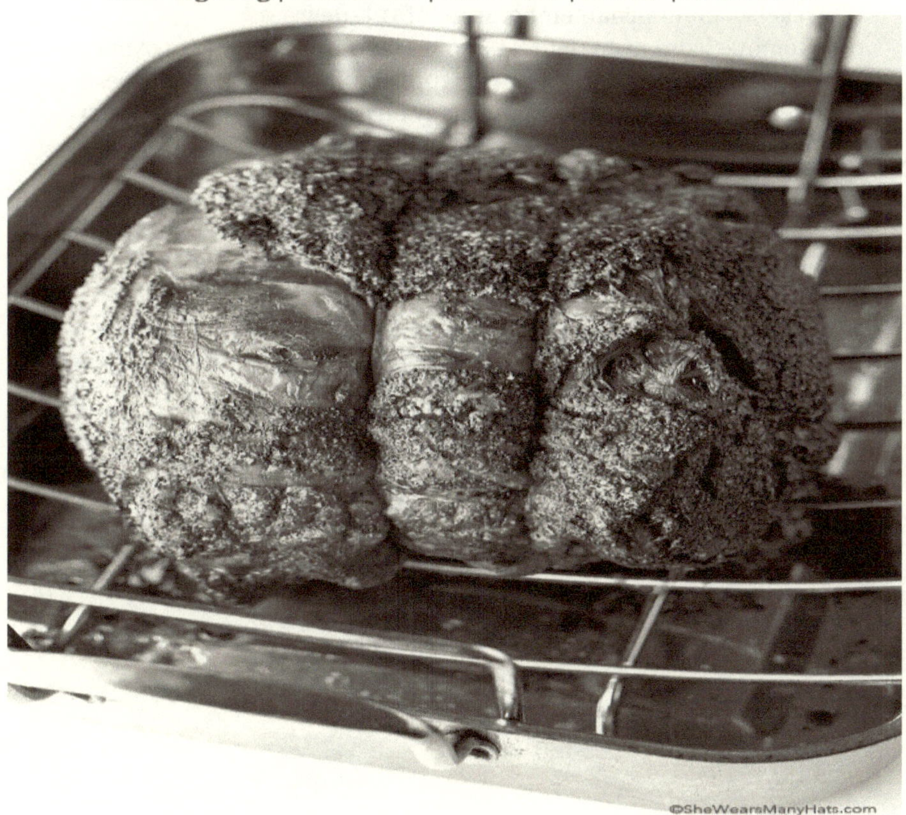

A fabulous main entree perfect for the holidays or other special occasions that is easier to prepare than you think.

Ingredients

- standing rib roast (2-7 ribs)
- kosher salt
- ground black pepper

Instructions

1. Preheat oven to 475-degrees F. Place rack in bottom 3rd of oven.
2. Liberally coat roast with salt and pepper. Place roast in roasting pan and let come to room temperature; about an hour.

3   Place roast in oven and cook at 475-degrees F for 30 minutes in bottom 3rd of oven.
4   Reduce heat to 300-degrees F; cook for 30 minutes.
5   Reduce heat again to 275-degrees F; continue cooking until it reaches an internal temperature of 125-degrees F.
6   Remove from oven; let rest about 15-20 minutes. Carry over cooking will continue; internal temperature should reach 135-degrees F for medium rare. Cut and remove any strings before slicing to serve.

NOTES

- If time permits, liberally coat roast with salt and pepper; place on a rack, situated inside of a baking sheet or roasting pan; place in refrigerator for up to 3 days.
- Overall cook time is approximate and will depend on size of roast.
- Regarding servings size, depending on the roast, estimate about 1 rib per 2 people

Double dark chocolate caramel brownies {paleo, vegan}

Prep Time: 10 minutes // Cook Time: 40 minutes

Yield: 9 brownies

Category: dessert

Thanksgiving | Christmas | New Year | Easter | Halloween

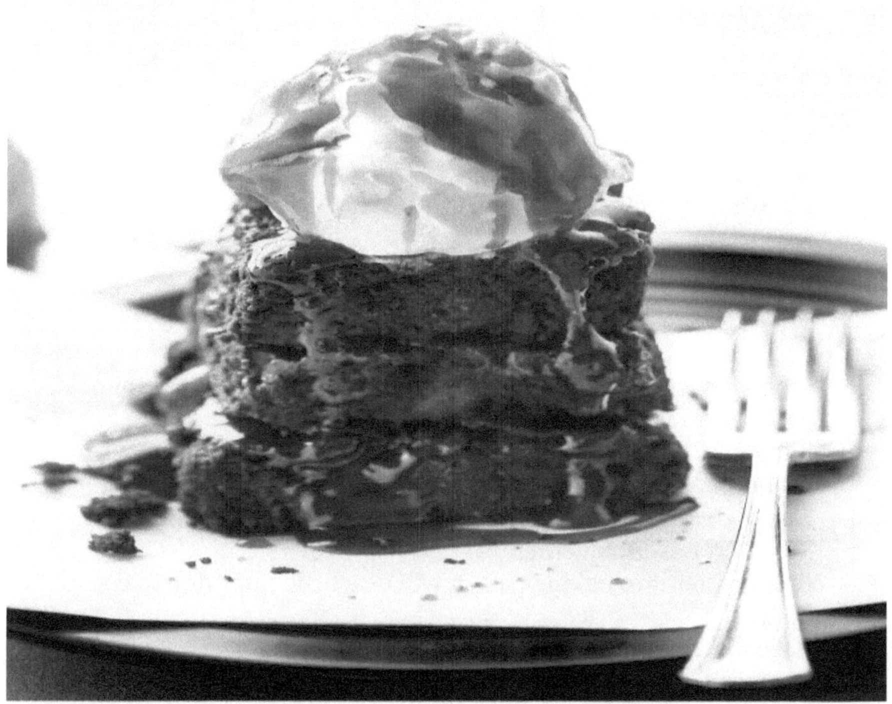

A vegan brownie recipe with dairy free salted caramel sauce, these fudgy dark chocolate brownies are also paleo and gluten free. The best healthier brownie with a superfood ingredient – cacao powder.

Ingredients

- 8x8 pan and parchment paper
- 1 cup almond flour
- 1/2 cup sifted coconut flour
- 1/2 cup cocoa powder or cacao powder

- 1 cup coconut palm sugar
- 2/3 cup pumpkin puree
- 1 cup dark chocolate chips or chunks
- w2 tsp distilled vinegar or other acidic liquid (lemon juice, apple cider vineger, etc.)
- w2 tsp vanilla
- 1 tbsp baking powder
- 1 tsp baking soda
- 1/2 c plus 1 tbsp coconut oil (about 8–9 tbsp total)
- 1/2 cup almond milk or other vegan milk of choice
- dash of salt

For the vegan salted caramel

You'll only use about half of this batch for the brownies

- 1/2 cup Coconut Palm Sugar
- 1/4 cup Agave or maple syrup
- 1.5 to 2 tbsp. Naturally refined Coconut Oil
- 1/2 – 1 tsp. sea salt
- 1/2 cup coconut milk

Instructions

1. Preheat oven to 350F. Line a 8×8 baking dish with parchment paper. I cut it to it fits.
2. Sift your flours together in one bowl.
3. Add in the rest of your dry ingredients. Mix together.
4. Next, add in your wet ingredients into different sections of the bowl.
5. Mix GENTLY all together.
6. Press batter into baking pan. It will be a little thick due to coconut flour.
7. Bake for 28-30 minutes.
8. Remove from oven, then let cool.
9. Once, cool enough, place in fridge to set the brownies before slicing.
10. While brownies are in fridge, make the salted caramel sauce.

Vegan Salted Caramel Sauce

1. In a small saucepan, mix the coconut sugar, agave, and coconut oil, and salt. Heat over medium heat, stirring to evenly melt the agave or maple syrup and coconut oil.
2. When sugar starts to soft boil (bubble), set the timer for two minutes. Stir the mixture once or twice during these two minutes.

3   Carefully stir in the coconut milk until it is mixed in and continue to heat until sauce returns to a low simmer.

4   Simmer low for 25-35 minutes. Stirring ever so often to get the caramel from the bottom of the pan. It will start to turn a darker amber color. The mixture will be soft and will continue to bubble a little bit during this whole process. NOTE: The longer you simmer it, the thicker the sauce will become when cooled.

5   Once it can coat the back of a wooden spoon (a thin coating), remove from heat and let it cool.

6   This is where it will thicken. Then store it in a covered glass container. Cool for 10 -12 minutes, stir, then you can place it covered in the fridge, if you are not using it right away. you can store it in fridge for up to two weeks. Makes around 3/4c to 1 cup.

7   Remove brownies from fridge, pour half of the caramel sauce on top or keep for individual slices. You will probably only use half the caramel so keep it in fridge for later uses. Like my caramelized apple bake

8   NOTE: Reheat the refrigerated caramel sauce in microwave for 30 to 40 seconds if you are wanting to use it again.

Serving Size: 1 brownieCalories: 300Sugar: 24.2gSodium: 257.4mgFat: 19.5gSaturated Fat: 10.7gCarbohydrates: 32.6gFiber: 5.5gProtein: 4.5gCholesterol: 0mg

NOTES

- The key to making these brownies set is refrigerating them a bit after you have removed them from the oven and they have cooled a bit.
- Store in fridge after cutting as well. These can also be frozen if you want to eat later.
- You will need the coconut oil to be a liquid.
- Once baked, set the pan in the fridge to "set" the brownies. You can make the caramel sauce when they are in the fridge.
- If you don't have cacao powder, just use unsweetened cocoa powder; both are great!

Mandarin-Roasted Turkey

Prep Time 15 minutes // Cook Time 45 minutes

Servings 4 -5

Course: Main Course

Paleo, Whole , Dairy Free, Gluten Free

I didn't host Thanksgiving, so we didn't get to enjoy turkey leftovers. I love to make turkey soup, so roasting a turkey was a must! I live in the Mandarin capital of California, so I wanted to make sure to use them in this recipe!

Ingredients

- 1 turkey (whatever size you like. Mine was about 10-12 pounds)
- mandarin oranges, cut in half
- 1/2 cup salt
- Herbes de Provence
- 1/4 cup ghee/Coconut oil

Instructions

1. Remove giblets from turkey. Set turkey in a large dish (I used a 9×13 pan), and generously cover with salt on all sides. Cover with plastic wrap and place in fridge overnight.
2. The next day, preheat oven to 425 degrees and baste the turkey in melted butter all over, then sprinkle with Herbes de Provence. Squeeze the mandarins over the turkey to give it a little flavor.
3. Place the mandarins inside the cavity. Place, breast side down, in roasting pan for about 25 minutes, then turn turkey over.
4. Make sure there are still herbs on the breast. If not, go ahead and sprinkle some more.
5. Bake in oven until internal temp reaches about 165 degrees. For me, it was about another 2 hours.
6. Cover lightly with a piece of aluminum foil and let sit for 20-30 minutes before carving.

Optional gravy recipe:

1. Take the drippings from the pan and put them in a saucepan. Add 1-2 cups water, depending on how salty it is.
2. When the salt level is right for you, turn heat to medium and cook until beginning to boil.
3. Get about 3 TBSP tapioca flour in a bowl, and add a couple TBSP of water.

4   Stir until the flour is dissolved and is milky white.
5   Add into the gravy, and continue to boil for a few more minutes, until starting to thicken. Superman said it was the best gravy he's ever had!

Butterflied Leg of Lamb and Spiced Pumpkin

Prep Time: 30 minutes | Cook Time 35 minutes

Thanksgiving | Christmas | New Year

Serves 4-6

Even if you don't love lamb, you'll love this easy recipe! So delicious and it pairs perfectly with the sweet and warm pumpkin!

Ingredients

- 5 lb. butterfly leg of lamb
- 1 teaspoon fine salt
- 1 teaspoon ground black pepper
- ½ onion slices
- 1 lemon sliced
- 3 tablespoons avocado oil
- 2 pumpkins (I used 1 kabocha squash, 1 sugar pumpkin)
  1 teaspoons garam masala
- 1 teaspoon cinnamon
- 1 teaspoon fine salt
- 2 teaspoons coconut aminos
- 3 tablespoons avocado oil

Instructions

1. First marinate the lamb ahead of time, I recommend 4 hours to overnight.
2. Toss the lamb with onion, lemon, salt, pepper and oil in a large bowl and store in the fridge overnight.
3. When you're ready to begin cooking the pumpkin remove the lamb from the fridge so it comes to room temperature. Pre-heat the oven to 400F.
4. In the meantime, halve your pumpkins carefully and use a spoon to scoop out the seeds.
5. Then cut side down on the cutting board and slice them into thin arches, 1/8-1/4 inch thick.
6. Distribute the pumpkin over two sheet pans.
7. Sprinkle the seasonings evenly over all of them, the coconut aminos and the oil.
8. Toss well to coat all the pieces then lay them flat on the sheet pans again, making sure the pieces are not overlapping.

9. Place in the oven on the middle and bottom rack. Roast for 35 minutes.
10. When there is 15 minutes left on the timer, begin cooking your lamb.
11. Heat a large cast iron skillet over medium heat, when it comes to temperature add in 1 tablespoon of fat.
12. Add the butterfly leg of lamb and sear 2 minutes. Then flip over. Add the lemon and onion to the skillet too. Sear another two minutes.
13. Open the oven, move on of the sheet pans to the top rack, and put your skillet with the lamb on the middle rack.(If your oven doesn't have 3 racks, let the pumpkin finish cooking before making the lamb).
14. Cook everything in the oven for 12-15 minutes, or until the lamb reads 145F internal temp.
15. Remove from the oven and let the lamb rest for 5 minutes before slicing

Bacon Wrapped Meatloaf

(Keto, Paleo, Whole , Egg Free)

Prep Time: 10 mins // Cook Time: 50 mins

Thanksgiving | Christmas | New Year | Halloween

Yield: 6

Method: Bake

Serving size: 6

Once you taste and see how lovely this keto, Whole compliant, paleo bacon wrapped meatloaf cooks up, you'll say it's Holiday table worthy. A great, affordable option that is a total crowd pleaser. From young children to adults, you can't go wrong with this dish.

A beautiful egg free bacon wrapped meatloaf!

Ingredients

- ½ large red onion, minced
- 4 cloves garlic, minced
- 1 ½– 2 pounds ground beef 85% lean
- 1/2 tablespoon fine Himalayan salt (1 1/2 teaspoon)
- 1 teaspoon ground black pepper
- 2 teaspoons garlic powder
- 1 teaspoon onion powder
- 2 teaspoons ground mustard seed
- 2 tablespoons flax meal
- 2 tablespoons red wine vinegar
- 2 tablespoons avocado oil
- ½ pound bacon, 7-8 slices

Instructions

1. Pre-heat oven to 400F. Line a sheet pan with parchment paper.
2. Combine the onion, garlic, beef and all of the seasonings in a large bowl. Mix thoroughly to combine.
3. Add in the flax meal, red wine vinegar, and avocado oil, mix again until thoroughly combined.
4. Shape the meat into a log on the sheet pan about 8 inches long and 3-4 inches tall. Move it to the side. Lay your bacon slices down on the center of the sheet pan, line them up so they overlap one an another ¼ of an inch.

5. Lay the meatloaf log in the center of the bacon then starting at the same end where you finished laying the bacon, bring the bacon slices up, wrapping the meatloaf in them, creating a seam at the top. Make sure you're wrapping it tightly.
6. Quickly flip it over to the bacon seam is on the bottom. Fix your bacon slices if you need to, make sure there are no gaps in it.
7. Place the sheet pan in the oven and bake for 50 minutes, or until the bacon is browned and crispy. Let it cool for 10 minutes.
8. Slice the meatloaf in slices the width of the bacon slices. Serve right away.
9. Store leftover in an airtight container for up to a week. Heat the slices in a skillet over medium heat until warm.
10. Substitutions: If you can't do flaxseed you may omit it and use 1 large egg. To make this AIP, omit the ground mustard, black pepper, and flax seed. Add in 1 teaspoon ground ginger instead and use 1 teaspoon of coconut flour.

Calories: 354, Fat: 27g, Carbohydrates: 2.5g, Fiber: 0.9g, Protein: 23.9g

Low Carb Sweet Potato Casserole

(Whole , Paleo, Keto, Dairy/Nut/Coconut Free)

Prep Time: 10 mins // Cook Time: 50 mins

Thanksgiving | Christmas | New Year | Easter | Halloween

Yield: 8

Method: bake

Cuisine: American

Thanksgiving: Made Whole

Let's be honest, Thanksgiving isn't going to be a day that revolved around macros or diets, keto or paleo. It's about spending time with your loved ones. Celebrating everything we are thankful for.

That being said, you don't want to throw your whole way of eating out the window. For one, you want to actually ENJOY the day, and that means feeling great.

Secondly, life goes on after Thanksgiving. Some folks brave the scary Black Friday crowds. Some have mountains of dishes and a house to clean. Others get on an airplane and fly home

A great low carb option for sweet potato casserole!

Ingredients

VEGETABLE PREP

- 1 large head cauliflower (4 cups diced)
- 1 large sweet potato (1 cup small diced)
- 1 cup pumpkin puree
- 4 cloves garlic
- 1 teaspoon salt
- ½ cup bone broth

MIX TO MASH

- 1/3 cup primal kitchen mayo
- 2 large eggs
- ½ teaspoon salt
- 1 tsp cinnamon
- 1 tsp garam masala (see notes)
- ¼ nutmeg

CARAMELIZED BACON

- 4 slices bacon
- 3 tablespoons coconut aminos

Instructions

1. Steam/ simmer the cauliflower and sweet potato with the garlic cloves in a pot with a tight fitting lid until they are fork tender. Or you can throw everything in the pressure cooker and set to low for8 minutes.
2. Heat the oven to 350F.
3. Add all of the cauliflower, sweet potato, garlic and broth to the bowl of your stand mixer (or a large bowl and use a hand mixer). Add in the pumpkin and mix with the paddle attachment on medium low speed.
4. While it mixes add in the mayo, then the eggs one at a time. Add in the seasoning. Mix until thick and well combined. Taste it! Add more salt or spice as you see fit.
5. Use a spatula to scrape all of the mash into a lightly greased casserole dish. Smooth out the top with a spatula and bake for 25 minutes.
6. In the time, cut the bacon slices into 1 inch pieces. Toss in a small bowl with 2 tablespoons coconut aminos. When the 25 minutes are up, open the oven and carefully distribute the bacon over the top of the sweet potato. Try to lay the pieces flat and so they don't overlap.
7. Sprinkle the remaining tablespoon of coconut aminos all over the stop. Close the oven, set to 400F. Bake for another 25 minutes.
8. Remove from the oven, let it rest a few minutes. Garnish with fresh herbs if you like. Serve with a large spoon or spatula.

Calories: 173, Fat: 115g, Carbohydrates: 13.9g, Fiber: 4.3g, Protein: 5.3g

Aunt Jen's Pumpkin Bread/Muffins

Dairy-Free, Gluten-Free, Soy-Free

Prep Time 10 minutes// Cook Time 15 minutes

Thanksgiving | Christmas | New Year | Easter | Halloween

Makes: 6

Ingredients

- 1 1/2 cups White Sugar
- 1 3/4 cups Flour (I used Gluten Free King Arthur 1:1 flour)
- 1 tsp. Baking Soda
- 1/4 tsp. Salt
- 1/2 tsp. Cinnamon
- 1/4 tsp. Nutmeg
- 1/2 cup Oil (I used Canola)
- 2 Eggs
- 1/3 cup Water
- 1 cup 100% Pure Pumpkin (I used canned)

Nuts Optional - Mixed In or Just on Top

Instructions

4. Preheat oven to 350 degrees. Add all of the dry ingredients into a large bowl. Whisk together to ensure they are mixed up.
5. Add the liquids, mix with hand mixer until combined.
6. Pour into greased pans (I sprayed with Avocado Oil) mini loaf pans, large muffin pans, cupcake tins, etc. Bake until done. The toothpick should come out clean.

Bacon & Egg Breakfast Wraps with Avocado

Prep Time 5 minutes // Cook Time 10 minutes

Thanksgiving | Christmas | New Year | Easter

Servings 2

Calories 469kcal

These breakfast wraps are filled with bacon & eggs, cheddar cheese, avocado and salsa. This low carb and super easy recipe will keep you full all morning.

Ingredients

- 2 Almost Zero Carb Wraps
- 3 slices bacon cooked
- 2 large eggs
- 1/2 cup grated cheddar cheese
- 1/2 avocado sliced
- 1/4 cup salsa
- salt and pepper to taste

Instructions

1. Cook the bacon in the pan until crisp. Remove, cut in half and set aside. Pour out all but 2 teaspoons of bacon fat. Slice the avocado.
2. In a small bowl, beat the eggs and half of the cheddar cheese cheese with a fork. Cook the scrambled eggs to your liking and remove from the pan. Season with salt and pepper.
3. Place the wraps into the hot pan over medium heat (I had to overlap mine just a bit in the middle).
4. Divide the scrambled eggs and place them on 1/2 of each wrap, not going past the middle. Add the avocado, bacon and remaining cheese. Add 1 tablespoon of water to the pan and cover quickly with a lid.
5. Leave covered for 1-2 minutes or until the cheese has melted and the bottom of the wraps have browned a bit. Serve with salsa.

Calories: 469kcal | Carbohydrates: 4g | Protein: 27g | Fat: 38g | Fiber: 1g

Creamy Root Vegetable Soup

Prep Time: 10 minutes // Cook Time: 35 minutes

Thanksgiving | Christmas | Halloween

Course: Side Dish, Soup

Servings: 6 cups

AIP, Dairy-Free, Gluten-Free, Grain-Free, Low-Carb, Paleo, Vegan

This creamy root vegetable soup is both comforting and nourishing!
You wouldn't know it's paleo, low carb, dairy-free, gluten-free, and
AIP friendly!

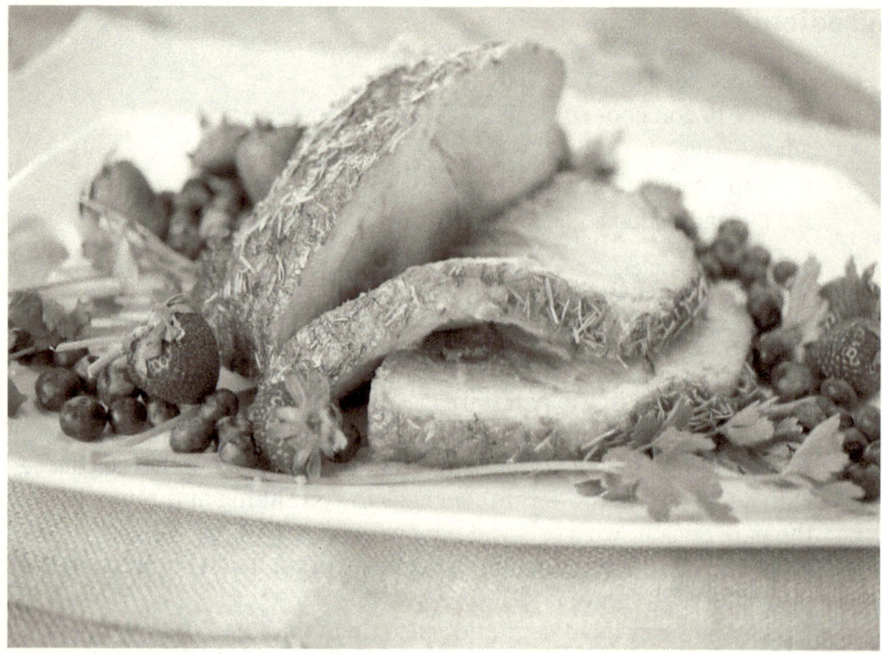

Ingredients

- 1 Tbsp ghee/Coconut oil (for AIP)
- 1 onion (medium; chopped)
- cloves garlic (minced)
- apples (approx 1 1/2 cups; peeled & diced--use chayote squash for
  low carb)
- 1 1/2 cups celery root (peeled and diced)
- 1 cup parsnip (peeled & diced--use turnip for low carb)
- 1 cup Japanese sweet potato (peeled & diced--see notes for low carb)
- cups water

- 2 cups homemade stock
- 2 tsp oregano
- 1 tsp salt (or to taste)
- 1 cup full-fat coconut milk

Instructions

1. Preheat a large stockpot over medium heat.
2. Add fat and let it heat a bit.
3. Saute onion for 2-3 minutes until soft.
4. Add garlic, cook for one minute and add all diced root vegetables. Saute until starting to soften, about 10 minutes, stirring occasionally.
5. Add the water, stock, oregano, and salt.
6. Bring to a simmer and cook until all root vegetables are fork tender.
7. Using a blender or food processor, puree the soup along with the coconut milk until smooth. Taste and add additional salt if desired.

Notes

1. Coconut oil or olive oil can be used instead of ghee for AIP.
2. See this post for some great tips on peeling garlic.
3. For low carb, sub chayote squash or peeled zucchini for the apples.
4. Use turnip instead of parsnip for low carb.
5. Any variety of sweet potatoes can be used instead of Japanese, however it will change the color. Use more celery root, or use radishes or jerusalem artichoke for low carb.
6. You can use chicken or vegetable stock –

Slow Cooker Ham (Paleo and AIP)

Prep Time: 5 minutes // Cook Time: 6 hours

Thanksgiving | Christmas | Halloween

Yield: 8

Method: Slow Cooker

Ingredients

- 1 4-6 lb Ham Roast
- 1/4 cup Honey
- 1/2 cup Orange Juice
- 2 tsp Dried Rosemary
- 3 tbs Coconut Oil
- zest of 1 Orange
- 1 tbs Apple Cider Vinegar

Instructions

- Place ham in slow cooker.
- Put the rest of the ingredients on the ham.
- Cook on low for 4-6 hours.

Notes

You can use a spiral sliced ham for this but I'd keep the cooking time more on the low end (closer to 4 hours or even less) as the slices allow it to cook faster and get dried out faster.

Crispy Creamy Green Bean Casserole

Prep Time: 15 mins//Cook Time: 45 mins

Thanksgiving | Christmas | New Year

Yield: 6

Category: Main

Method: Oven

Cuisine: Thanksgiving

At some point when you are making a number of substitutions for a dish, like this keto friendly, dairy free, green bean casserole, you just have to take some creative liberty. You might be hesitant about the ingredient list, but this healthy green bean casserole blows the traditional versions out of the water!

Ingredients

THE GREEN BEANS

- 2 pounds green beans,fresh, trimmed
- 5 slices sugar free bacon
- 2 cups sliced cremini mushrooms
- THE ONIONS
- 2 cups sliced onion, 1/4 inch thick slices
- ¼ teaspoon salt
- 3 tablespoons avocado oil

THE SAUCE

- 2 cups diced cauliflower
- 1 cup coconut milk
- 4 cloves garlic
- ½ teaspoon salt
- ½ teaspoon black pepper
- ¼ teaspoon nutmeg
- 1 tablespoon nutritional yeast
- 3 egg yolks

Instructions

1. Pre-heat your oven to 400F.

2. Combine the cauliflower, garlic cloves and coconut milk in a sauce pot, cover with a lid and heat over medium heat. Cook here until the cauliflower is fork tender.
3. In the meantime, arrange your green beans side by side vertically in rows, in one flat layer over 2 sheet pans.
4. Sprinkle the mushrooms all over. Cut the bacon into small pieces and distribute it evenly over all of the veggies. Sprinkle with a pinch of salt. Roast for 20 minutes, middle and bottom rack. Rotate the pans after 10 minutes.
5. In the meantime heat a large skillet over medium heat. Add in the oil then the onions. Sprinkle in the salt. Use tongs or forks to gently toss. Then cover with a tight fitting lid.
6. Stir every 5 minutes until green beans are ready. They will begin to get tender, then translucent, then browned and finally soft and sweet with some toasty bits!
7. By now the cauliflower should be soft. Carefully transfer all the contents of the sauce pot to a blender. Add in the seasoning and the nutritional yeast. Blend on high until smooth, add in a little bit of water or broth if needed. Then add in the egg yolk one at a time until fully combined
8. When the green beans are ready remove them from the oven. They will be browned and crunchy, try not to eat them all.
9. Arrange them in a casserole dish, I like to arrange them in little bunches with the greens beans (with the mushrooms and bacon pieces) all facing the same way, makes it easier to serve. Pick a few pieces of bacon out and set them aside.
10. Pour the cream sauce all over the green beans and use a spatula to spread it out. Then top with the caramelized onions and those bacon pieces you set aside.
11. Pop the casserole in the oven and bake for 20 minutes.
12. Remove from the oven, and serve!

Nutrition

Serving Size: 1/6 Recipe, Calories: 190, Fat: 10.4g, Carbohydrates: 15.1g, Fiber: 6.5g, Protein: 9g

Herbed Slow-Cooked Lamb Shanks

Prep time: 30 mins //Cook time: 180 mins

Thanksgiving | Christmas | New Year | Easter | Halloween

Ingredients

- 4-5 large lamb shanks (I managed to squeeze 5 large shanks into my le Creuset)
- 1 tablespoon fresh rosemary (chopped)
- 1 tablespoon fresh thyme (finely chopped)
- sea salt
- 1 teaspoon dried oregano or marjoram
- 1 teaspoon ground cinnamon
- 1 tablespoon happy fat (I used beef tallow)
- 2 large carrots, quartered and diced
- 4 sticks celery, diced
- 1 large leek, washed and finely sliced
- 2 large onions,finely chopped
- 2 garlic cloves, peeled and chopped
- 2 tablespoon fresh rosemary, finely chopped
- 2 tablespoon apple cider vinegar
- 100 ml verjuice or white wine
- 6 anchovy fillets
- 250 mls bone broth
- Handful flat-leaf parsley (chopped)

Instructions

1. Heat your oven to 180°C/350°F. I start by washing and chopping all my vegetables. Put aside in a large bowl.
2. Throw chopped rosemary, thyme, dried oregano, cinnamon, and salt into your mortar and pestle. Give it a good bash. Rub the shanks in this mixture, pressing it in well. I find the best way to do this is to place your meat in a large plastic bag.
3. Pour the herb mixture in and give it a good shake, ensuring each shank gets a good covering of the rub.
4. Heat a thick-bottomed casserole pan, add your fat of choice and – when the fat has melted – brown the meat on all sides in batches and remove from the pan.
5. Add the carrot, celery, onions, leek and garlic along with the extra chopped rosemary and a pinch of salt and sweat them until softened (about ten minutes).
6. Add the apple cider vinegar and allow it to reduce to a syrup.

7. Pour in the verjuice and allow to simmer for a couple of minutes.
8. Add the anchovies and then add the bone broth. Shake the pan and return the lamb to the casserole. Shimmy the shanks around to get a nice fit.
9. Bring to the boil, put on the lid and pop in the oven for 2 – 2½ hours to work its magic. Then, remove the lid and cook for a further half an hour.
10. If you want to take the meat off the bone, now is the time to do so. Carefully remove your shanks from the casserole. Using two forks, gently pull the meat from the bone. It should fall away. Once shredded, the meat can be returned to the casserole. I also take care to ensure I have removed all the marrow from the bones and pop that back into the dish.
11. Taste for seasoning. Finally, stir in a handful of roughly chopped fresh parsley.

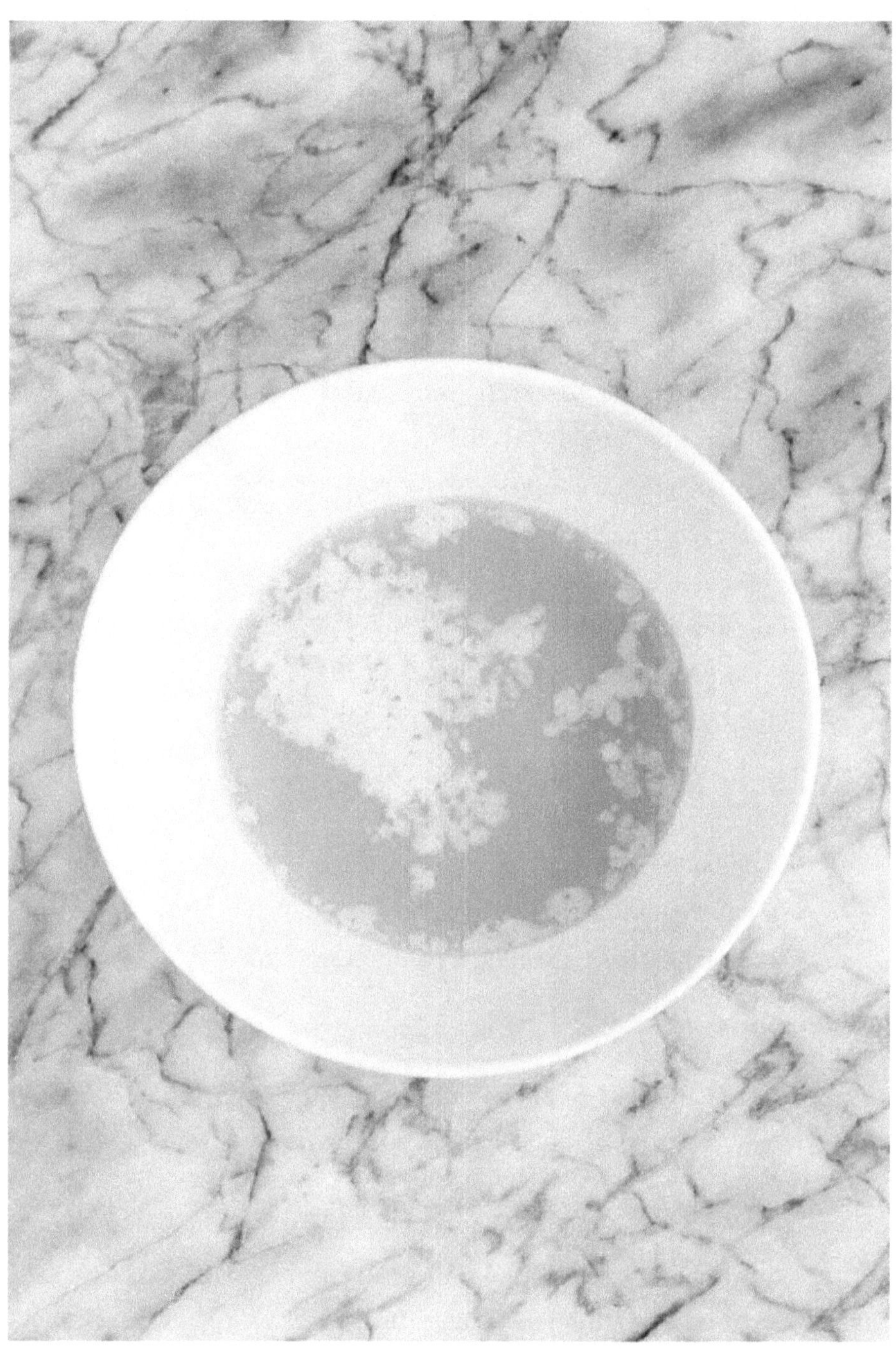

Creamy Garlic Chicken

Prep Time: 10 Mins // Cook Time: 15 Mins

Thanksgiving | Christmas | New Year | Easter | Halloween

Yield: 3

Serving Size: 1/3 Recipe

Recipe Type: Main dish

Ingredients

- 3 medium chicken breasts (approx 1.3lbs)
- 1 ¾ teaspoon fine salt, divided
- 1 teaspoon ground cumin
- ½ teaspoon black pepper
- ½ teaspoon mustard powder
- ¼ teaspoon nutmeg
- 2 tablespoons olive oil
- 5 cloves garlic, sliced
- 3 sprigs thyme, leaves only
- 1 lemon
- ½ cup bone broth
- 1 ½ cup cashew cream (see post for nut free)
- 9 ounces spiralized zucchini, 2 medium squash

Instructions

1. Put your chicken breasts on a plate and pat them dry. Then season with 1 ½ teaspoon salt, cumin, pepper, mustard powder, and nutmeg.
2. Pour the 1 tablespoon olive oil in your skillet. Add the chicken and sear without moving for 4 minutes. Flip over, cover the skillet and cook another 3 minutes. Remove the chicken from the skillet and set on a cutting board.
3. Add the remaining oil to the skillet. Add in the garlic and thyme. Sauté until the garlic is toasted and very aromatic. Add in the lemon

juice and bone broth, bring to quick simmer. Gently stir to deglaze the skillet.

4. Add in the cashew cream and remaining salt, gently stir as it begins to thicken, 3-4 minutes, then remove from heat. Slice the chicken breasts, and serve one breast with 3 ounces of zoodles on each plate. Cover with ½ a cup of creamy garlic sauce. Enjoy!

5. You can also add the zoodles and sliced chicken back into the skillet and mix it all together before serving, but folks might fight over who got more sauce

CALORIES: 391, FAT: 19.1g, CARBOHYDRATES: 8.8g, FIBER: 2.2g, PROTEIN: 41.1g

Crock Pot Turkey Bolognese Sauce

Prep Time: 10 mins || Cook Time: 6 hrs

Thanksgiving | Christmas

Serves: 6

Cooking Type: Baking

Course: Main dish

For an easy weeknight dinner serve this crock pot turkey Bolognese sauce with zucchini noodles.

Ingredients

For sauce

- 1 28- ounce can organic tomato puree
- 1 6- ounce can organic tomato paste
- 1/2 cup chicken stock
- 1 tablespoon olive oil
- 2 teaspoons Italian herb blend
- 1 teaspoon sea salt
- 1/2 teaspoon pepper
- 1/8 teaspoon crushed red pepper flakes
- 3 cloves garlic minced
- 2 small carrots diced
- 1 small onion diced
- 1 pound ground turkey

For zucchini noodles

- 3- 6 medium zucchini

Instructions

To make sauce

1. Add all sauce ingredients except turkey to slow cooker and stir to combine.
2. Cut ground turkey into cubes, add to slow cooker, and cover with sauce. Do not stir.
3. Cook on low for 6-8 hours.
4. Once the sauce is done, use a potato masher to break up the ground turkey into small chunks.

To make zucchini noodles

1	Spiralize zucchini (1/2 - 1 medium zucchini per serving).
2	Heat one tablespoon olive oil in large frying pan over medium heat. Cook zucchini until warmed through but still firm, about 3 minutes.

Notes

Variations: serve the sauce over roasted spaghetti squash or other spiralized veggie noodles.

Calories: 231kcal | Carbohydrates: 27g | Protein: 24g | Fat: 5g | Cholesterol: 42mg | Sodium: 743mg | Potassium: 1602mg | Fiber: 6g | Sugar: 15g | Vitamin A: 4840IU | Vitamin C: 49.6mg | Calcium: 84mg | Iron: 4.7mg

Cilantro-Lime Salmon Recipe

Prep: 10 min || Cook: 20 min

Thanksgiving | Christmas | New Year | Easter | Halloween

Cooking Type: Oven

Serves: 2

Ingredients

- 2 salmon fillets
- 1/2 cup coconut oil, melted
- Juice and zest of 2 limes, and then slice the limes
- 2 garlic cloves, minced
- 1/4 cup fresh cilantro, roughly chopped + more for garnish
- Sea salt and freshly ground black pepper

Instructions

1. Preheat oven to 375 F.
2. Place the lime slices in baking a dish, then season the salmon fillets to taste with sea salt and freshly ground black pepper on both sides; place fish on top of the lime slices.
3. In a bowl, combine lime juice, lime zest, cilantro, garlic, and coconut oil.
4. Pour the mixture over the salmon and place in the oven.
5. Cook 15 to 20 minutes, or until salmon reaches desired doneness.
6. Let the salmon rest 2 to 3 minutes, and serve topped with fresh cilantro and fresh lime slices.

Protein: 50g / 21%, Carbs: 8g / 3%, Fat: 82g / 76%

Cheeseburger Casserole with Bacon

Prep Time 20 minutes // Cook Time 35 minutes

Thanksgiving | Christmas | New Year | Easter | Halloween

Main Course

Servings 12 people

Calories 587kcal

Need a simple ground beef casserole to feed your family or friends? They will love this easy burger casserole with bacon.

Ingredients

- 2 pounds ground beef
- 2 cloves large garlic
- 1/2 teaspoon onion powder
- 1 pound no sugar bacon cooked and chopped
- 8 eggs see note
- 1 can tomato paste 6 ounces
- 1 cup coconut heavy cream
- 1/2 teaspoon salt
- 1/4 teaspoon ground pepper
- 12 ounces grated Vegan cheddar cheese divided

Instructions

1. Brown ground beef with garlic and onion powder.
2. Drain excess grease, then spread beef on bottom of 9×13-inch casserole pan.
3. Stir bacon pieces into cooked beef.
4. In medium bowl, whisk together eggs, tomato paste, coconut heavy cream, salt, and pepper until well combined.
5. Stir 8 ounces grated cheese into egg mixture.
6. Pour egg mixture over beef and bacon.
7. Top with remaining 4 ounces of grated cheese.
8. Bake at 350°F for 30-35 minutes or until golden brown on top.

Notes

If you want a less eggy casserole, reduce eggs and add more beef. Mushrooms, onions, and pickles are great add-ins!

Total Fat 49g 75%|Saturated Fat 22g 110%|Cholesterol 244mg
81%|Sodium 735mg 31%|Potassium 505mg 14%|Total Carbohydrates 4g
1%|Sugars 2g|Protein 29g 58%|Vitamin A 19.3%|Vitamin C 4.1%|Calcium
25.5%|Iron 15.3%

Cajun Chicken Eggroll in a Bowl

Prep Time: 5 mins // Cook Time: 20 mins

Thanksgiving | Christmas | New Year

Servings: 4 servings

Ingredients

- 1 Pound Boneless Skinless Chicken Breast cut into pieces
- 10 Cups Chopped Cabbage 1 medium head
- 2 Tablespoons Yellow Mustard
- 2 Teaspoons Creole Seasoning
- 1 Teaspoon Smoked Paprika
- 1 Teaspoon Garlic Salt
- 1 1/2 Teaspoon Italian Seasoning
- 1 Teaspoon Chili Powder
- 1/2 Teaspoon Liquid Smoke
- 3/4 Cup Water
- Snipped Fresh Cilantro optional

Instructions

1. In a large skillet, brown chicken.
2. When chicken is cooked through, add chopped cabbage, all seasonings, and water.
3. Stir, while allowing to cook for 5-10 minutes, or until cabbage is wilted to your desired tenderness.

Calories - 160 Fat - 2 grams Carbs - 13.4 Fiber - 5.9 Net Carbs - 7.5 Protein - 24.1

Bacon-Wrapped Whole Turkey with Herb Butter

Prep Time: 20 min // Cook Time: 3 hr, 30

Thanksgiving | Christmas | Halloween

Serves 12

Bacon-wrapped anything is amazing, so enjoy this turkey during the holidays!

Ingredients

- 1 (5kg) whole turkey, insides removed
- 10-15 slices of bacon
- 2 onions, quartered
- 4 carrots, roughly chopped
- 3 celery stalks, roughly chopped
- 1 lb potatoes, cut small
- 3 garlic cloves
- 1/4 cup chicken broth
- Salt and pepper

Herb Butter

- 2 tbsp. freshly chopped sage
- 2 tbsp. freshly chopped thyme
- 1/2 cup coconut oil, room temperature
- 1 garlic clove, minced
- Salt and pepper

Gravy

- Turkey pan drippings
- 1 tbsp. flour (or more if necessary)
- 1/2 cup white wine
- Salt and pepper

Instructions

1. To make the herb butter, combine the coconut oil, sage, thyme, and garlic. Season with salt and pepper.

Turkey

2. Preheat oven to 425F.

3. Pat your turkey dry. Season with salt and pepper, along with your veggies and garlic. Stuff the cavity with as much of the veggies as you can. Add the rest of the veggies to the bottom of the pan and add the turkey on top. Pour broth into the bottom of a baking dish. Rub the herb butter all over the turkey until completely coated (making sure to get under the skin!!!).
4. Bake, uncovered, for 30 minutes.
5. Reduce oven to 350F. and baste. Cook for 1 hour 30 minutes, basting every 30 minutes if necessary.
6. Remove from oven and drape with bacon slices. Cook for another 1 hour, basting every 20-30 minutes. The turkey is done when it reaches 160F. You may need more or less time depending on the size of your turkey!
7. Remove turkey from pan and cover with aluminum foil: allowing to rest for 30 minutes or longer to get those juices moving! Slice and serve!

Gravy

1. To make the gravy, pour pan drippings into a large pan and heat over medium. Pour in white wine and simmer for a couple of minutes.
2. Add the flour and whisk constantly until thickened (I generally cook my sauces for about 5 minutes to really get that flour taste out.)

Notes

Cook time may vary, but if you find you add your bacon too early and it is beginning to burn, just cover it in aluminum foil.

CREAMY GARLIC PARMESAN MUSHROOMS

Prep Time: 5 Minutes // Cook Time: 5 Minutes

Thanksgiving | Christmas | New Year | Easter | Halloween

Servings: 4

Side Dishes

Creamy Garlic Parmesan Mushrooms are sautéed in a coconut oil garlic until tender and then tossed in the most AMAZING creamy parmesan sauce. These are great as a side, on top of meat or eaten by themselves and ready in under 10 minutes!

Ingredients

- 2 Tablespoons Coconut oil
- 1 Tablespoon olive oil
- 8 Ounces white mushrooms whole or sliced to preference
- 2 cloves garlic minced
- 1/2 cup Coconut heavy cream
- 1/4 cup grated Vegan parmesan cheese
- 2 ounces Paleo cream cheese softened
- 1 teaspoon italian seasoning
- 1/2 teaspoon salt
- 1/4 teaspoon pepper
- fresh chopped parsley for garnish

Instructions

1. In a medium sized skilletover medium high heat add the coconut oil and olive oil. Add the mushrooms and garlic and saute until tender.
2. Add the heavy cream, parmesan cheese, cream cheese, italian seasoning, salt and pepper. Stir with the mushrooms and heat until the sauce is bubbly and smooth.
3. Serve immediately and garnish with fresh parsley.

Calories 276Calories from Fat 243, Fat 27g42%, Saturated Fat 15g75%, Cholesterol 77mg26%, Sodium 496mg21%, Potassium 222mg6%, Carbohydrates 4g1%, Fiber 1g4%, Sugar 2g2%, Protein 6g12%, Vitamin A 857IU17%, Vitamin C 2mg2%, Calcium 113mg11%, Iron 1mg6%

Spaghetti Squash Au Gratin with Bacon

Prep Time: 15 mins // Cook Time: 50 mins

Thanksgiving | Christmas | New Year | Easter | Halloween

Servings 10

Growing up, I loved potatoes au gratin and scalloped potatoes. That was even the highly processed, "just add water and powdered cheese" varieties that came from a box. In the constant search to replace those starchy potatoes we all love, spaghetti squash has proven to be a worthy opponent.

Ingredients

- 1 Large Spaghetti Squash
- 2 Tbs. Olive Oil
- 2 Tbs. Coconut oil
- 2 Cloves Garlic – Minced
- 1 Small Onion – Thinly Sliced
- Salt and Pepper – To Taste
- 8 Slices Bacon – Cooked Crisp and Crumbled
- 1 ½ Cup Sour Cream
- 2 Cups vegan Cheddar Cheese – Shredded
- ¼ Cup Vegan Parmesan Cheese – Grated

Instructions

1. Preheat oven to 400° Line a rimmed baking sheet with aluminum foil.Cut spaghetti squash in half lengthwise and scrape out the seeds.
2. Drizzle olive oil over spaghetti squash, sprinkle with salt and pepper, and place cut side down on baking sheet. Bake 30 minutes. Remove from oven and allow to cool.
3. While the squash is roasting, heat a medium sauté pan over medium heat. To the pan add coconut oil, garlic, onions, salt and pepper. Cook until onions are lightly caramelized
4. Once the squash has cooled, use a fork to scrape the flesh into a large mixing bowl. To the bowl, add onions, bacon, sour cream, cheddar cheese, and Parmesan cheese.
5. Mix until all ingredients are well incorporated. Transfer to a casserole dish.
6. Reduce oven temperature to 350° Bake for an additional 20 minutes.

Calories – 280, Protein – 16 g, Carbs – 8 net g, Fat – 5 g

Bacon Green Bean Casserole

Prep Time: 20 minutes // Cook Time: 20 minutes

Thanksgiving | Christmas | New Year | Easter | Halloween

Yield: 6 servings

Category: Side Dish

Serving Size: ¾ Cup (~115g)

Try this easy low carb keto bacon green bean casserole! It will make the perfect low carb keto side dish for dinner, Thanksgiving, Christmas or a dinner party!

Ingredients

- 60g (~1 cup) finely crushed pork rinds
- 1 tsp minced onion
- ¾ tsp salt, divided
- 4 slices bacon
- 12 oz green beans, ends trimmed
- ¼ cup sauvignon blanc
- 2 tbsp bacon grease
- 2 tsp dried parsley
- ½ cup chicken broth
- 4 oz Coconut cream cheese, softened, cut into small pieces
- 1 ½ oz shredded Vegan cheddar cheese
- 1 ½ oz shredded Vegan mozzarella cheese
- 1 tsp dijon mustard
- ⅛ tsp black pepper

Instructions

1. Preheat oven to 350 degrees and grease 8×8 baking pan with nonstick cooking spray.
2. To a small bowl, whisk together crushed pork rinds, minced onion, and ¼ tsp salt. Set aside.
3. Fry bacon in a large pan until crisp. Transfer bacon to paper towel-lined plate to remove excess grease. Reserve 2 tbsp bacon grease. Crumble bacon using hands. Set aside.
4. Steam green beans over high heat in a steamer basket for 3-4 minutes. Transfer steamed green beans to a large bowl, add crumbled bacon, and mix until well-combined.
5. To a large pot over medium heat, add sauvignon blanc, reserved bacon grease, and dried parsley, and cook until smell of wine has dissipated about 2-3 minutes. Add chicken broth and stir.

6. Add cream cheese and allow to melt fully before mixing in shredded cheddar, shredded mozzarella, mustard, ½ tsp salt, and pepper. Continue to cook, stirring frequently, until all ingredients are melted together and well-incorporated.
7. To the bowl of green beans and crumbled bacon, pour in cheese mixture and mix until combined. Transfer to the prepared baking pan, top with crushed pork rind mixture, and bake until edges are golden brown and bubbling, about 18-20 minutes. Serve hot and enjoy!

Allergy

- Low Carb and Keto: One serving contains only 4.9 grams of net carbs!
- Nut Free: This keto green bean casserole is nut-free and safe to consume for those with nut allergies or nut intolerances.
- Egg Free: This Thanksgiving casserole does not include any eggs.
- Coconut Free: There are no coconut products in this keto casserole recipe.
- Gluten Free and Grain Free: This is a gluten-free dish, as well as being free from grains, and is safe to consume for those with Celiac disease.
- Sugar Free: This keto casserole recipe is made without any added sugar or sweeteners.

Spicy Sausage and Cheddar Stuffing

Prep Time: 10 mins // Cook Time: 45 mins

Course: Side Dish

Thanksgiving | Christmas | New Year | Easter | Halloween

Servings: 16 servings

Calories: 311 kcal

1 serving = about 1/2 cup

GLUTEN FREE

This Keto Sausage and Bread Stuffing is going to be the star of your Thanksgiving table! Made with my famous low carb cheesy skillet bread and plenty of sausage, it's full of traditional stuffing flavor without all the carbs.

Ingredients

- 1 recipe Cheesy Skillet Bread **check below**
- 12 ounces spicy Italian sausage
- 1 cup diced celery
- 1/2 cup diced onion
- 2 garlic cloves minced
- 1 teaspoon dried sage
- 1/2 teaspoon kosher salt
- 1/4 teaspoon black pepper
- 1/2 cup low sodium chicken broth
- 2 large eggs
- 1/4 cup coconut heavy cream

Instructions

1. A day or two in advance, make the skillet bread and cube into 1/2 inch pieces. Preheat oven to 200F.
2. Spread bread cubes on a large baking sheet and bake 2 to 3 hours, until well dried and crisp. Let sit out overnight to continue to dry.
3. Heat a large skillet over medium heat and add sausage; sauté until just cooked through, about 6 minutes, breaking up large chunks with a wooden spoon.

4. Using a slotted spoon, transfer sausage to a large bowl. Add celery, onion, garlic, sage, salt and pepper to skillet and sauté until tender, about 5 minutes. Add to sausage.
5. Preheat oven to 350F and coconut oil a large 13x9 inch glass baking dish. Add cubed bread to sausage mixture. Add chicken broth and toss to combine.
6. In a medium bowl, whisk eggs with cream and pour over mixture in bowl. Toss until well combined and transfer to prepared baking dish. Bake 35 minutes, uncovered, until top is crusty and browned.

Calories 311Calories from Fat 238, Fat 26.4g41%, Carbohydrates 6g2%, Fiber 3.2g13%, Protein 11.5g23%

Cheesy Skillet Bread

Prep Time: 10 mins // Cook Time: 16 mins

Thanksgiving | Christmas | New Year | Easter | Halloween

Calories: 357 kcal

Servings: 10

(1 slice (1/10th of bread)

Easy low carb skillet bread with a wonderful crust of cheddar cheese. This keto bread recipe is perfect with soups and stews, and makes the BEST low carb Thanksgiving stuffing!

Ingredients

- 1 tbsp coconut oil for the skillet
- 2 cups almond flour
- 1/2 cup flax seed meal
- 2 tsp baking powder
- 1/2 tsp salt
- 1 & 1/2 cups shredded Vegan Cheddar cheese divided
- 3 large eggs lightly beaen
- 1/2 cup coconut oil melted
- 3/4 cup almond milk

Instructions

1. Preheat oven to 425F. Add 1 tbsp coconut oil to a 10-inch oven-proof skillet and place in oven.
2. In a large bowl, whisk together almond flour, flax seed meal, baking powder, salt and 1 cup of the shredded cheddar cheese.
3. Stir in the eggs, melted coconut oil and almond milk until thoroughly combined.
4. Remove hot skillet from oven (remember to put on your oven mitts), and swirl coconut oil to coat sides.
5. Pour batter into pan and smooth the top. Sprinkle with remaining 1/2 cup cheddar.
6. Bake 16 to 20 minutes, or until browned around the edges and set through the middle. Cheese on top should be nicely browned.
7. Remove and let cool 15 minutes.

Serves 10. Each serving has 7.2 g of carbs and 4 g of fiberCheesy Skillet Bread

Calories 357Calories from Fat 276, Fat 30.63g47%,
Carbohydrates 7.9g3%, Fiber 4.77g19%, Protein 12.48g25%

Parmesan Roasted Brussels Sprouts with Bacon

Course Side Dish

Thanksgiving | Christmas | New Year | Easter | Halloween

Servings 6

Parmesan Roasted Brussels Sprouts with Bacon are roasted to perfection, with crispy bacon and lots of Parmesan cheese.

Ingredients

- 2 lbs Brussels fresh sprouts
- 2 tablespoons olive oil
- 6 pieces cooked bacon roughly chopped
- 1/2 cup grated vegan Parmesan
- 1 1/2 teaspoon kosher Salt
- 1 teaspoon fresh ground pepper

Instructions

1. Preheat oven to 400 degrees
2. Cut the ends off the brussels sprouts then cut them in half if they are large.
3. Place them in a large bowl and add the olive oil, half of the Parmesan and salt and pepper and toss them.
4. Then place them on a baking sheet and roast for 20-25 minutes stirring about halfway.
5. Add the bacon and the rest of the Parmesan and additional salt and pepper if needed serve.

Garlic Roasted Green Beans and Mushrooms

Prep Time: 10 mins // Cook Time: 25 mins

Thanksgiving | Christmas | New Year | Easter | Halloween

Servings: 4 servings

Side Dish

Delicious Garlic Roasted Green Beans and Mushrooms are a delicious and healthy side dish. This side is simple to make with just a few fresh vegetables and pantry staples.

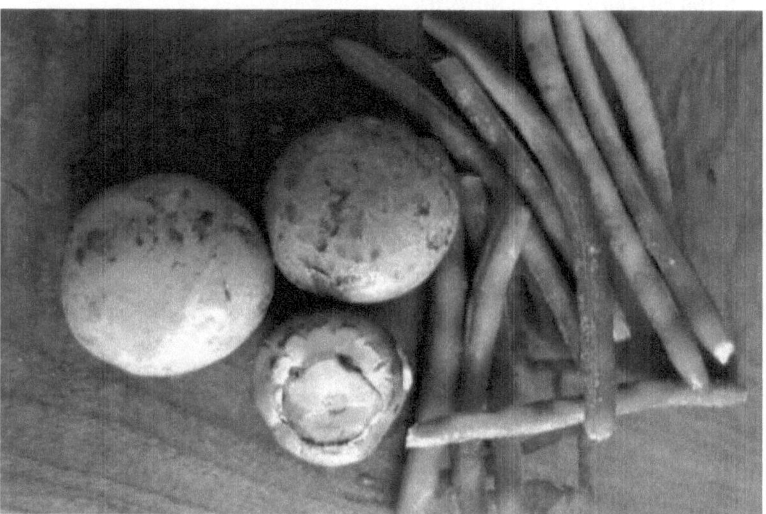

Ingredients

- 2 cups sliced fresh mushrooms
- 2 cups fresh green beans
- 1/4 cup olive oil
- 2 teaspoons minced garlic
- 1 teaspoon freshly ground sea salt
- 1 teaspoon freshly ground pepper

Instructions

1. Preheat oven to 400.
2. Wash and slice mushrooms and green beans.
3. Combine oil, garlic, salt and pepper in a separate bowl.
4. Pour over the mushrooms and green beans and gently stir until vegetables are thoroughly coated.

5. Place on baking sheet and bake for 20-25 minutes. Serve warm.

Garlic Herb Bacon Wrapped Turkey Breast

Prep Time 10 minutes // Cook Time 1 hour

Course Main Course

Thanksgiving | Christmas | New Year | Easter | Halloween

Servings 4 people

Calories 910 kcal

Dairy free, Egg free, Gluten free, Peanut free

This bacon wrapped turkey breast is covered in a balsamic garlic herb rub then wrapped in a bacon weave for a flavorful, juicy turkey recipe.

Ingredients

- 3 tbsp balsamic vinegar
- 2 tbsp olive oil
- 6 sprigs fresh rosemary divided
- 6 sprigs fresh thyme divided
- 2 tbsp steak seasoning
- 6 cloves garlic crushed
- 4 lb boneless, skinless turkey breast
- 10 slices bacon

Instructions

1. Preheat the oven to 400°F.
2. Whisk the balsamic vinegar & olive oil together in a small bowl.
3. Chop 4 sprigs of rosemary & 4 springs of thyme, add to the bowl with the steak seasoning & crushed garlic.

Brush this mixture over the turkey breast.

4. Place the two remaining sprigs of rosemary & thyme on top of the turkey.
5. Weave the bacon slices together over the turkey.
6. Tuck the bacon under the turkey.
7. Make sure the ends of the rosemary and thyme sprigs slightly stick out at the end for easy removal after the turkey has baked.
8. Place the bacon wrapped turkey on top of a wire rack on a foil-lined baking sheet.
9. Brush any extra herb rub on top of the bacon.
10. Place in the oven and bake for 1 hour (or until the turkey breast reaches 165° inside).

Beef Chili with Bacon in the Instant Pot

Serves: 10

Prep Time: 10 mins || Cook Time: 30 min

Thanksgiving | Christmas | New Year | Easter | Halloween

Course: Main dish

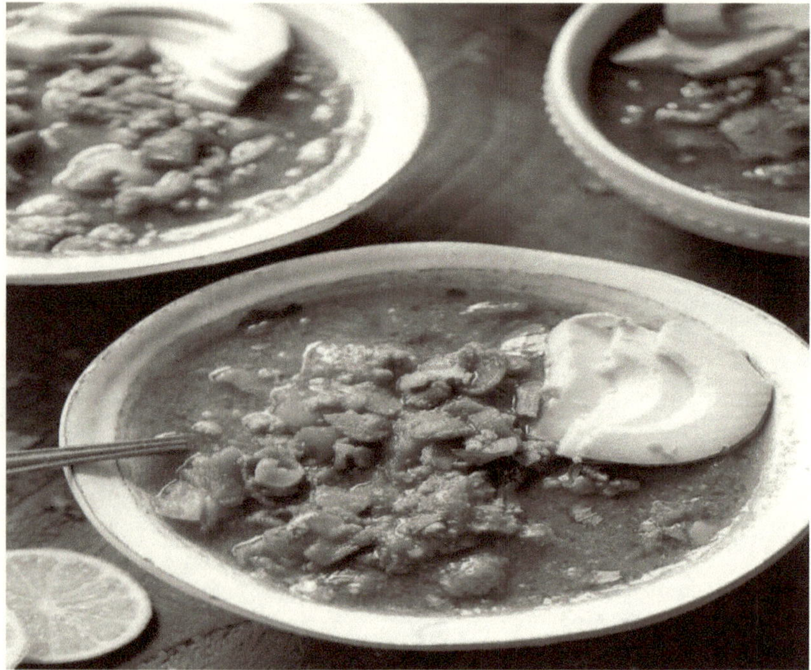

This easy instant pot beef chili is packed with everything you're craving! Savory ground beef and bacon, peppers, onions and garlic and the perfect spices. It's paleo, dairy-free, Whole compliant and keto friendly, delicious and family approved!

Ingredients

- 1 1/2 lbs ground beef grass fed
- 1/2 lb bacon nitrate free and sugar free for Whole foods, cut into pieces
- 1 medium onion chopped
- 1 large red bell pepper chopped
- 2 small jalapeno peppers seeded and minced
- 3 cloves garlic minced

- 28 oz can diced tomatoes
- 6 oz can tomato paste
- 12 oz bone broth beef flavored, homemade or purchased
- 1 tsp cumin
- 1 tsp smoked paprika
- 1 Tbsp chili powder
- 1/2 tsp chipotle powder
- 1 tsp fine grain sea salt
- Cilantro for garnish
- lime for garnish
- avocado sliced, for garnish

Instructions

1. Have all ingredients chopped and ready to go before beginning. Press "sauté" on the instant pot and once hot, cook bacon until crisp, stirring. Remove with slotted spoon and set aside.
2. Discard all but 1 tbsp bacon fat, then add beef and brown, stirring to break up lumps.
3. Once beef is 75% done, add veggies and sauté until tender. Press "cancel" and add remaining ingredients, place the lid on top and turn vent to seal, then cook on high pressure 10 mins (pot will take several minutes to heat up).
4. Once done, quick release the pressure, then add bacon back to chili, saving some for garnish.
5. Allow the chili to cool a few minutes before serving. Garnish with cilantro or other herbs plus extra bacon and avocado slices, and serve as is, over a sweet potato or with homemade tostones! Enjoy!

Calories: 313kcalFat: 23gSaturated fat: 8gCholesterol: 63mgSodium: 600mgPotassium: 625mgCarbohydrates: 9gFiber: 2gSugar: 5gProtein: 17gVitamin A: 1140%Vitamin C: 30.7%

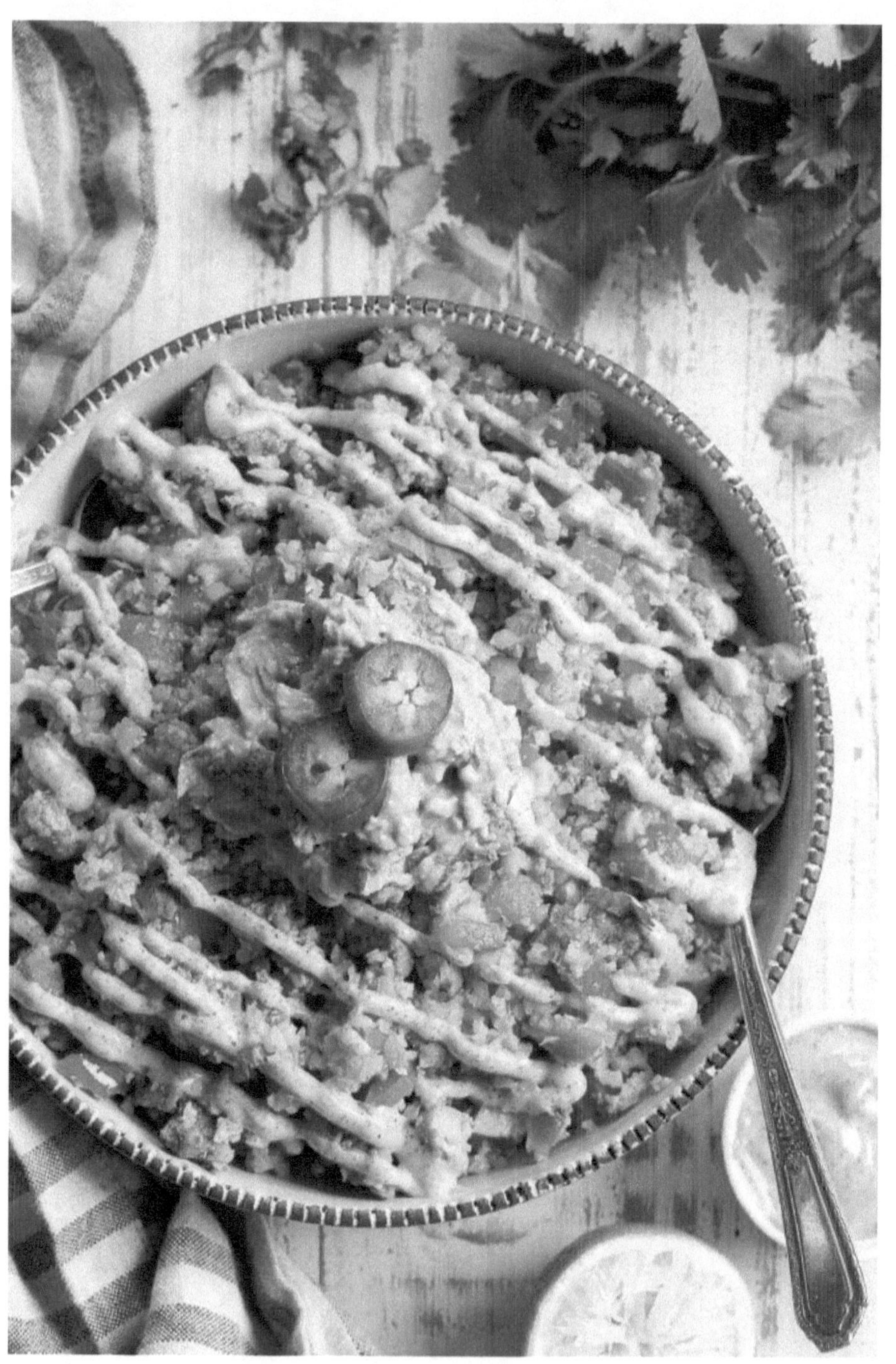

Mexican Cauliflower Fried Rice

Serves: 6

Prep Time: 15 mins || Cook Time: 15 mins

Thanksgiving | Christmas | New Year | Easter | Halloween

Cooking Type: Stove Top

Course: Main dish

This Mexican Cauliflower Rice is packed with veggies, protein, and lots of flavor and spice! It's topped with an easy guacamole and chipotle ranch sauce for a tasty, filling meal that's Paleo, Whole foods compliant and keto friendly.

Ingredients

- 12 oz riced cauliflower about 1 head, just shy of 4 cups
- 1 lb ground beef turkey, chicken, or pork
- 3 Tbsp cooking fat coconut oil, bacon fat, olive oil, ghee, divided
- 1/2 tsp fine grain sea salt
- 1/2 tsp onion powder
- 1/2 tsp garlic powder
- 1 tsp cumin
- 1 tsp chili powder
- generous dash chipotle pepper adjust to your taste or omit
- 1 red bell pepper diced
- 1 small yellow onion diced
- 3 garlic cloves minced
- 1 can chopped green chilis
- 1 jalapeno pepper seeds removed and minced
- Cilantro for garnish
- 1/2 cup homemade chipotle ranch dip
- 1 batch easy guac see below:

easy guac:

- 1 large ripe avocado or 2 small, mashed
- 2-3 Tbsp onion minced
- 1 clove garlic minced
- 1-2 Tbsp jalapeno peppers minced
- 1 1/2 Tbsp fresh lime juice
- 2 Tbsp chopped fresh cilantro plus more for garnish

Instructions

1. Prepare the chipotle ranch, cover and chill until ready to serve.
2. Heat a skillet over medium heat and add 1 Tbsp coconut oil.
3. Add ground meat to skillet and sprinkle with salt and spices. Once browned, add onion, pepper and stir, cook about 45 seconds until softened.
4. Add chopped green chilis, garlic, and jalapeno pepper and continue to cook another 45 seconds to heat through. Add cauli rice and stir to coat, then cover skillet for 30 seconds to soften cauliflower, remove from heat.
5. Before serving, mash together all the guac ingredients in a bowl. To serve fried rice, top with extra cilantro, chipotle ranch and guac. Enjoy!

Calories: 335kcalFat: 27gSaturated fat: 12gCholesterol: 53mgSodium: 273mgPotassium: 604mgCarbohydrates: 9gFiber: 4gSugar: 2gProtein: 15gVitamin A: 855%Vitamin C: 63.8%Calcium: 36%Iron: 2.3%

Crispy Paleo Chicken with Creamy Mushroom Sauce

{Whole, Keto}

Serves: 5

Prep Time: 10 mins || Cook Time: 35 min5

Thanksgiving | Christmas | New Year | Easter | Halloween

Cooking Type: Baking

Course: Main dish

This crispy paleo chicken with creamy mushroom sauce is made all in one skillet, packed with flavor, dairy free, paleo, keto and Whole compliant! Seasoned crispy skinned chicken thighs with a dairy free mushroom sauce that's perfect over cauliflower rice or with roasted and veggies

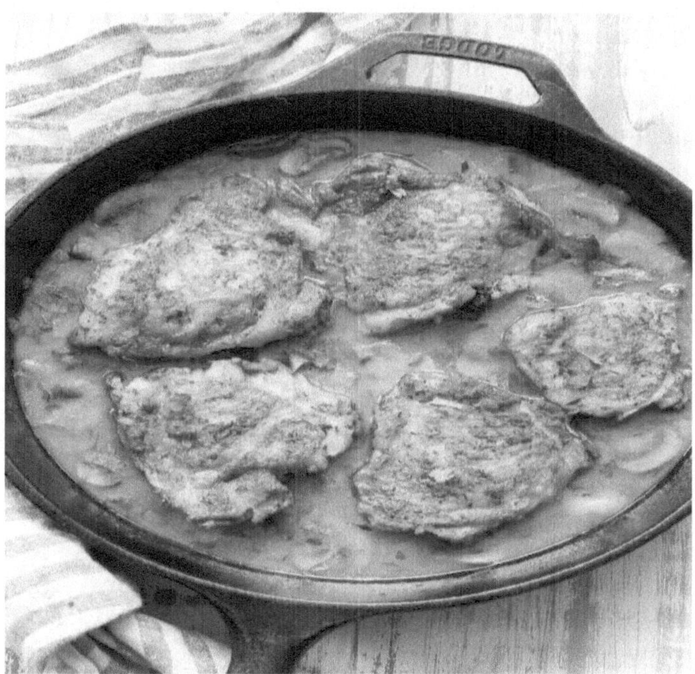

Ingredients

- 5-6 bone-in skin-on chicken thighs
- Sea salt and and pepper to season chicken
- 1 tsp dried sage

- 1/2 tsp dried thyme
- 3 Tbsp olive oil divided
- 8 oz white mushrooms washed and sliced
- 1/2 medium onion chopped (or 1 small)
- 2 cloves garlic minced
- 8 oz chicken bone broth
- Sea salt and pepper
- 1/4 cup full fat coconut milk blended prior to adding
- 2 tsp spicy brown mustard
- 2 tsp tapioca or arrowroot starch

Instructions

1. Preheat your oven to 400 degrees
2. Heat a large cast iron skillet (or any oven proof skillet) over med-high heat. Season chicken with salt, pepper, sage, and thyme, rubbing in seasonings to coat skin.
3. Add 2 Tbsp olive oil to skillet, then brown chicken in skillet on both sides - about 2-3 minutes per side.
4. Once browned, remove chicken from skillet to a plate and lower heat to medium, add 1 more tbsp ghee to melt.
5. Add onions and cook one minute until softened, then add mushrooms and garlic and continue to cook 3 minutes over med heat until softened. Season with salt and pepper to taste, stir in broth, and remove from heat.
6. Return chicken and any juices back to skillet, place skillet in preheated oven and bake 25 minutes, until cooked through, return skillet to stovetop.
7. Remove just the chicken from skillet with tongs to make the sauce. Whisk tapioca and mustard into coconut milk, then add to skillet and whisk to combine. Bring to a boil and allow to boil 2-3 minutes until thickened, stirring. Return chicken to skillet and serve with mushroom sauce. Enjoy! Serves 5-6.

Calories: 437kcalFat: 35gSaturated fat: 14gCholesterol: 164mgSodium: 127mgPotassium: 481mgCarbohydrates: 4gSugar: 1gProtein: 25gVitamin A: 115%Vitamin C: 2.1%Calcium: 18%Iron: 1.7%

Cranberry Pecan Cauliflower Rice Stuffing

Prep Time: 10 minutes // Cook Time: 30 minutes

Thanksgiving | Christmas | Halloween

Yield: 10 servings

Category: side dishes

This Cranberry Pecan Cauliflower Rice Low Carb Stuffing is the perfect keto Thanksgiving side dish. You can stuff it inside the turkey in place of traditional stuffing, or you can just serve it on the side.

Ingredients

- 3/4 cup raw pecans
- 2 tablespoons coconut oil
- 1 shallot, thinly sliced
- 1 cup chicken stock
- 6 cups riced cauliflower
- 2 sprigs fresh thyme
- 1 bay leaf
- 1 teaspoon sea salt
- 1/2 teaspoon ground black pepper
- 2 tablespoons chopped fresh flat-leaf parsley
- 1/2 cup grated Vegan Parmesan cheese
- 1/4 cup Low Carb Sugar Free Dried Cranberries (see Below)

Instructions

5. Preheat the oven to 350°F. Spread the pecans in a single layer on a rimmed baking sheet and roast them for 8 minutes.
6. Meanwhile, heat the coconut oil in a large skillet over medium heat. Add the shallot and sauté until it is soft and translucent.
7. Add the stock to the skillet and, using a rubber spatula, scrape and mix in any bits that are stuck to the bottom of the pan.
8. Add the riced cauliflower, thyme, bay leaf, salt, and pepper to the skillet. Cook for about 15 minutes, until all of the liquid has evaporated and the cauliflower is completely cooked and tender.
9. Remove the thyme sprigs and bay leaf and discard. Mix in the roasted pecans, Parmesan cheese, and dried cranberries. Taste and add more salt and pepper, if desired.
10. Store leftovers in the refrigerator for up to 1 week.

**Net Carbs Per Serving: 3.2g, Calories: 127 Fat: 10g
Carbohydrates: 5.5g Fiber: 2.3g Protein: 4.4g**

Sugar free low carb dried cranberries

Prep Time: 15 minutes // Cook Time: 4 hours

Thanksgiving | Christmas | New Year | Easter | Halloween

Yield: about 3 cups 1x

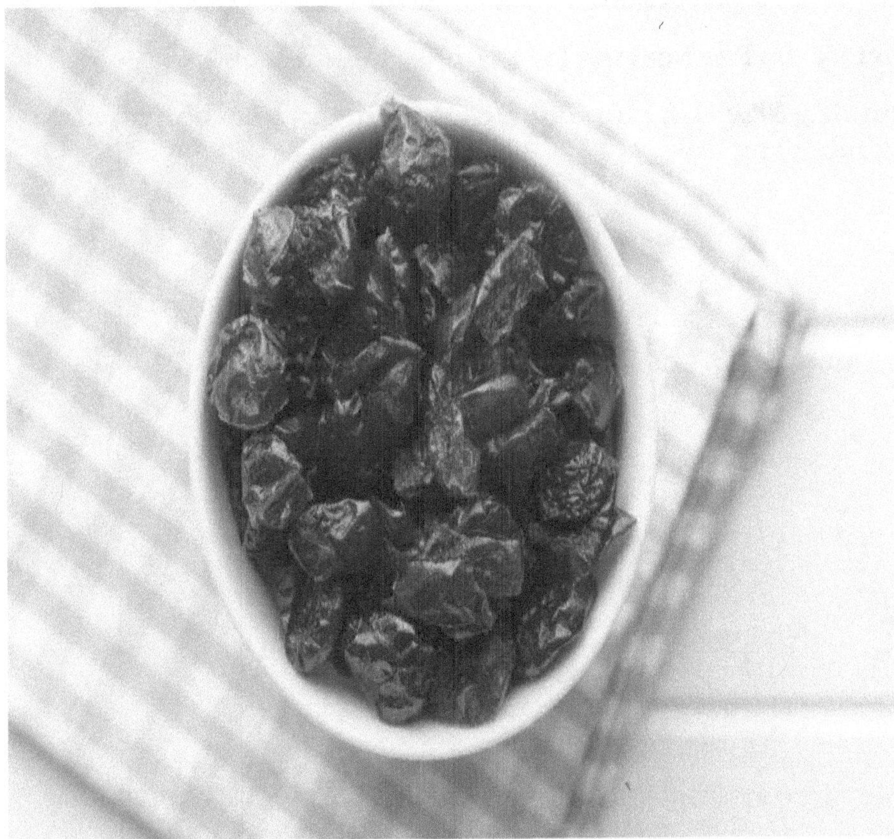

Ingredients

- 2 – 12 ounce bags fresh cranberries
- 1 cup granular erythritol or granular monk fruit sweetener (get it here)
- 3 tablespoons avocado oil
- 1/2 teaspoon pure orange extract

Instructions

1. Preheat the oven to 200°F. Line two rimmed baking sheets with parchment paper or a silicone baking mats.
2. Rinse and dry the cranberries and remove any browned or soft berries. Slice the cranberries in half and add them to a mixing bowl.
3. Add the sweetener, avocado oil, and orange extract, if using. Toss to evenly coat all of the berries.
4. Line the berries in single layers across the baking sheets.
5. Bake for 3 to 4 hours, rotating the racks half way through.

Net Carbs Per Serving (1/4 cup) – 5g

Serving Size: 1/4 cup Calories: 61 Fat: 3.5g Carbohydrates: 7g Fiber: 2g

Low-Carb & Keto Chocolate Pecan Pie

Keto, Gluten-free, Dairy-free, Sugar-free, Yeast-free, Corn-free, Grain-free, Low-Carb

Prep time: 20 mins // Cook time: 30 mins

Thanksgiving | Christmas | New Year | Easter | Halloween

Serves: 12

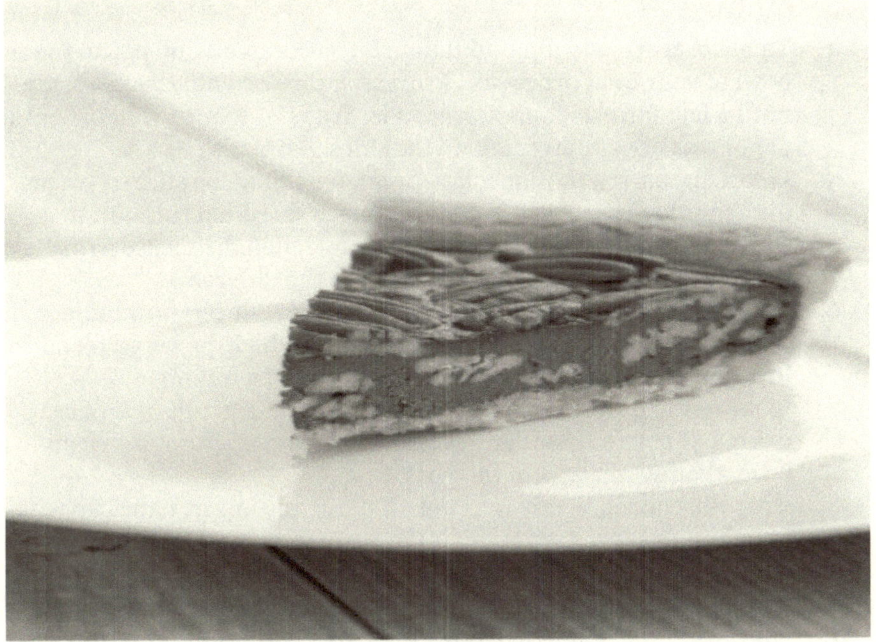

Ingredients

Grain-free, Paleo Pie Crust

- 2 cups (260 grams) ground blanched almonds
- ¼ teaspoon Himalayan rock salt
- 2 tablespoons suet or coconut oil
- 1 egg

Chocolate Pecan Pie Filling

- 6 tablespoons coconut oil, melted
- 3 oz. unsweetened dark chocolate squares (dairy-free), melted

- 3 eggs
- 1 cup finely shredded zucchini (255 grams freshly shredded, 195 grams once liquid has been wrung out)
- 1 ½ teaspoons pure vanilla extract
- ¾ teaspoon alcohol-free stevia
- 150 grams raw pecan halves, divided

Instructions

1. Preheat oven to 350F.
2. For a 9" pie, lightly oil a 9-inch pie pan with coconut oil. Set aside.
3. For 3" tarts, lightly oil six 3-inch circular tart pans with coconut oil. Set aside.
4. To make crust, add almond flour, salt, coconut oil and egg to the bowl of your food processor. Process and pulse with the "S" blade until a ball forms, about 30 seconds. Transfer to prepared pie or tart pan. Press dough, pressing up the sides. Set aside.
5. Before preparing the chocolate pecan pie filling, be sure to "wring out" shredded zucchini. To do this, place shredded zucchini in a clean cloth and wring out lightly. I've included the measurements of the wet and dry zucchini so you can see the difference.
6. Add melted coconut oil, dark chocolate, eggs, zucchini, vanilla and stevia to the bowl of your food processor or high-powered blender. Process or blend on high until smooth, about 1 minute.
7. Remove the processor bowl from the base and stir-in 75% of the pecans. If using a blender, transfer chocolate mixture to a clean bowl, then stir in 75% of the pecans.
8. Drop the chocolate mix into the prepared pie or tart pan. Top with remaining pecans.
9. For pie, bake in preheated oven for 35-40 minutes, until top is set and sides become golden. Once complete, allow to cool overnight.
10. For tarts, bake in preheated oven for 18-20 minutes, until top is set and sides become golden. Once complete, allow to cool for 1-hour before removing from tart pan. Tarts can be consumed immediately, or chilled overnight.
11. Serve with coconut whipped cream.
12. Makes six 3-inch tarts or one 9-inch pie.

Notes

Chocolate baking squares: I purchased these at the grocery store, in the baking isle. They were "Unsweetened Dark Chocolate Baking Squares"

Turkey Sausage, kale & Pumpkin Soup

Thanksgiving | Christmas | New Year | Easter | Halloween

Yield: Serves 8

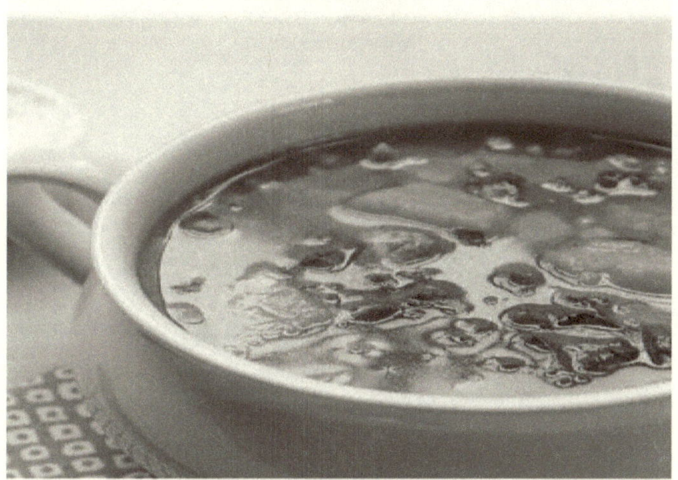

Ingredients

- 1 lb. sweet italian turkey sausage
- 1/2 cup chopped onion
- 3 cups chopped pumpkin or butternut squash
- 4 cups chopped kale
- 4 cups chicken broth
- 4 cups water

Instructions

1. Cook sausage in a medium sized saucepan. Add onions and sauté until translucent. Pour the broth and water into the saucepan and bring to a boil – reduce heat.
2. Add the kale and pumpkin and simmer until the pumpkin is soft, about 20 minutes.

Calories: 118, Fat: 6g, Carbohydrates: 5.5g net, Protein: 11g

Caramelized Balsamic Leek Turkey Hearts

Prep Time: 20 Mins || Cook Time: 20 Mins

Thanksgiving | Christmas | New Year | Easter | Halloween

Serves: 2 serve

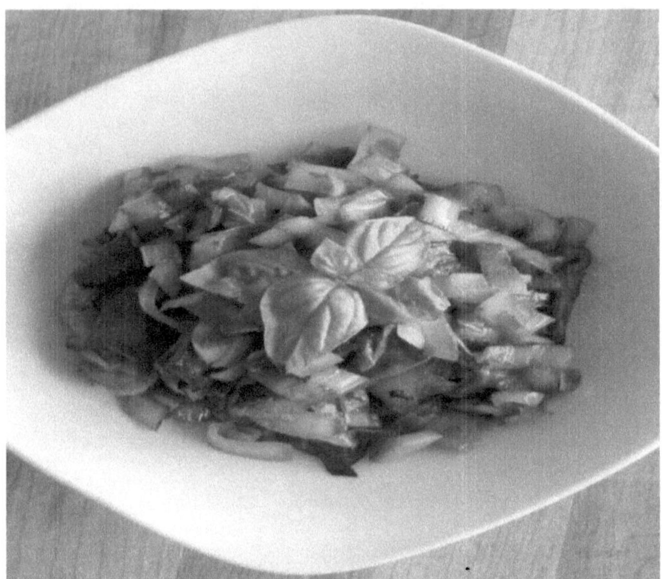

Ingredients

- 8 oz. turkey hearts
- 1/4 cup olive oil
- 3/4 tsp sea salt
- 2 tbsp balsamic vinegar
- 3 cups leek greens – chopped
- Fresh basil for garnish.

Instructions

1. Prepare turkey hearts by cutting each heart into fourths.
2. Heat 2 tbsp. olive oil in a large pan over medium heat, and once hot, add leeks and allow-ing them to cook until tender and fragrant.
3. Remove cooked leeks from the pan and set aside for later use, then add remalining 2tbsp olive oil to the pan, turning the heat to low.
4. Add prepared turkey hearts to the pan, sprinkle with remaining sea salt and cover, allow-ing them to cook for 2-3 minutes until no longer pink in the middle.

5. Add the cooked leeks back into the pan and deglaze the pan with the balsamic vinegar, quickly stirring to scrape up any crispy bits from the bottom of the pan, then take the pan off the heat and serve, topping with basil sprigs.

Recipe Notes

- The basil is optional, but highly recommended, as it adds an extra pop of flavor especially loved by the individuals I served this dish to
- If you don't have turkey hearts, chicken hearts work equally as great.

Easy Roast Turkey Breast Recipe

Serves: 8

Prep Time: 5 mins || Cook Time: 1 hr. 30 min

Thanksgiving | Christmas | New Year | Easter | Halloween

Course: Main dish

An easy roast turkey breast recipe for stress-free meals—from holidays to make-ahead dinners to healthy lunches.

Ingredients

- bone-in turkey breast halves 3-4 pounds each
- 2 tablespoons duck fat melted
- coarse ground sea salt to taste

Instructions

1. Preheat oven to 425 degrees.
2. Place turkey breast on a rimmed baking sheet, skin side up, and rub all over with duck fat. Season with salt.
3. Place in oven and reduce heat to 375 degrees. Roast until internal temperature reaches 165 degrees, about 1 to 1-1/2 hours.
4. Cover with foil and rest for 15 minutes before slicing.

Calories: 223kcal | Carbohydrates: 0g | Protein: 41g | Fat: 6g | Saturated Fat: 1g | Cholesterol: 107mg | Sodium: 397mg | Potassium: 467mg | Sugar: 0g | Vitamin A: 40IU | Calcium: 27mg | Iron: 1mg

Adobo Turkey Burgers

Prep Time: 5 mins // Cook Time: 10 mins

Thanksgiving | Christmas | New Year | Easter | Halloween

Yield: 6 burgers

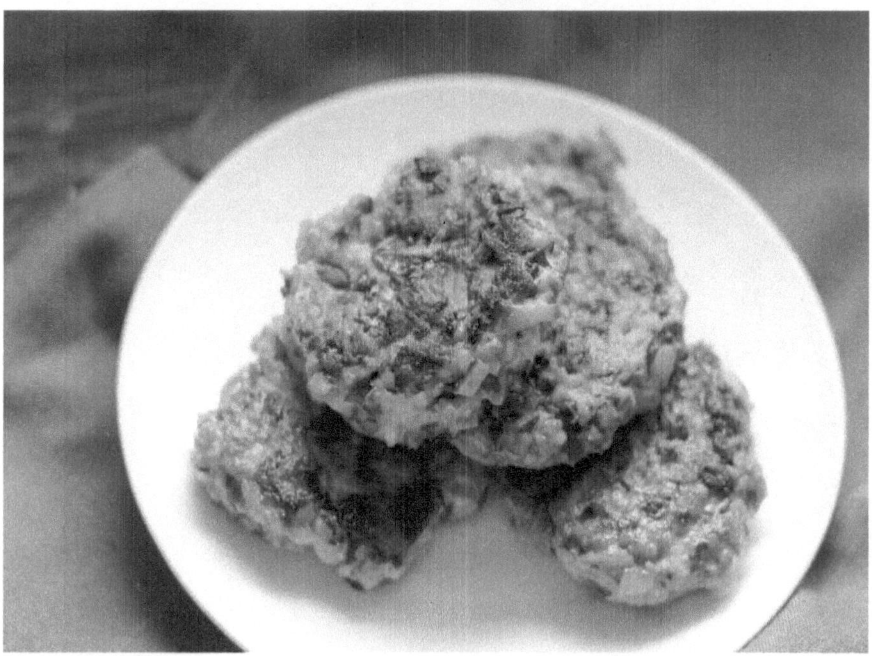

Ingredients

- Coconut oil
- 1 tsp garlic powder
- 1 tsp onion powder
- 1 tsp turmeric
- 1.5 tsp dried oregano
- 1lb ground turkey
- 1/4 cup red onion, finely diced
- 1 large handful of spinach, finely chopped (approximately 1 cup)
- 1/2 tsp Himalayan pink salt + more to taste

Instructions

1. Preheat oil over medium heat in a large cast iron skillet.
2. Mix ground chicken, red onion, spinach, and seasoning in a large bowl until well combined. Divide into 6 equal portions and form burger patties.

3. Cook burgers for 4-5 minutes per side or until it reaches an internal temperature of 165 degrees.
4. Serve warm over roasted vegetables, a bed of spinach, or in a lettuce wrap.

SIDE DISHES

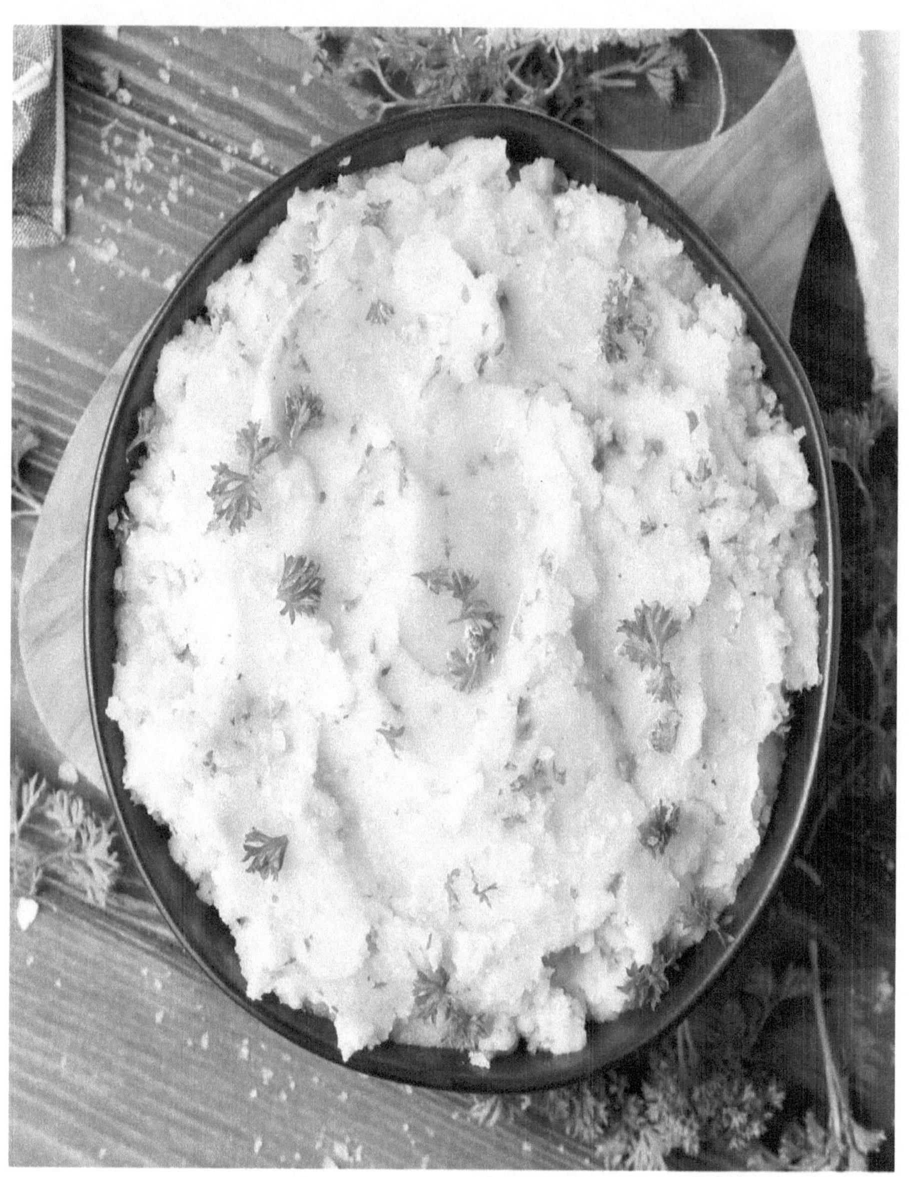

Dairy Free Garlic Mashed Potatoes

Prep Time: 5 Minutes Cook Time: 20 Minutes

Thanksgiving | Christmas | New Year | Easter | Halloween

Yield: 6

Serving Size: 8

These Dairy Free Garlic Mashed Potatoes don't need no stinkin' milk and butter to be great! Roasted garlic and parsley make these Whole Mashed Potatoes extra yummy! Use vegetable stock for Vegan Mashed Potatoes. A great side dish if you are on a special diet or not.

Ingredients

- 3 Lbs Russet Potatoes, (peeled, cubed)
- 1 Head of Roasted Garlic
- 1/2 teaspoon Sea Salt
- 1/4 teaspoon Fresh Cracked Pepper
- 1 Cup Chicken or Vegetable Stock*, (approximately)
- 1/4 Cup Chopped Fresh Parsley
- Ghee, (optional)

Instructions

1. Place (peeled,cubed) potatoes in large pot and fully cover with water. Bring to a boil. Boil until potatoes are tender when pricked with a fork. Time will vary depending on size of potatoes. Drain potatoes and transfer to large bowl.
2. Add garlic, salt and pepper. Add stock 1/4 cup at a time mixing in between additions with hand mixer. Continue to add stock until desired consistency (approximately 1 cup total). Mix in parsley.
3. Taste then salt/pepper as needed. Top with fresh parsley and ghee. Serve.

Notes

*If using vegetable stock, be sure it is the golden color stock and not red. Otherwise the mashed potatoes will have an interesting color.

Amount Per Serving

Calories 292, Total Fat 5g Saturated Fat 2g, Trans Fat 0g, Unsaturated Fat 3g, Cholesterol 27mg, Sodium 337mg, Carbohydrates 49g, Net Carbohydrates 0g, Fiber 5g, Sugar 3g,

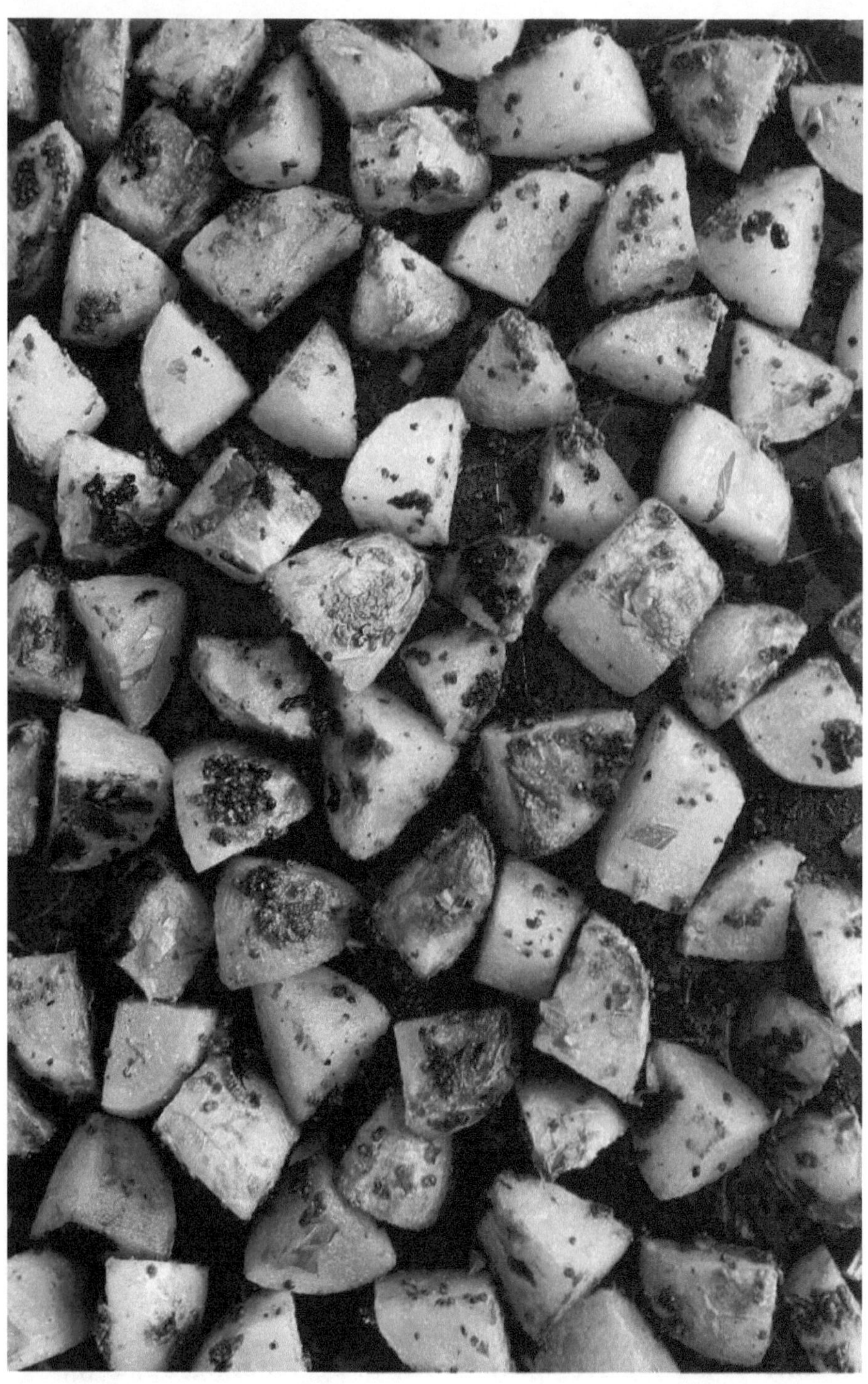

Mustard-Crusted Potatoes

These potatoes are a great side dish to any meal!

Ingredients

- 1/3 cup olive oil
- 1/3 cup Dijon mustard
- 1/3 cup whole-grain mustard
- Grated zest and juice of 2 lemons
- 4 garlic cloves minced
- 6 Yukon Gold potatoes peeled and quartered (about 6 cups)
- Kosher salt
- 1/2 fresh lemon cut into wedges
- Minced fresh flat-leaf parsley for garnish

Instructions

1. Preheat oven to 400 degrees F.
2. In a large bowl, whisk together the olive oil, mustards, lemon zest, lemon juice, and garlic. Add the potatoes and toss to coat with the mixture.
3. Spread the potatoes on a rimmed baking sheet and sprinkle generously with salt.
4. Bake for 30 minutes. Toss the potatoes, return to the oven, and bake for 15 minutes, or until the potatoes are a deep golden brown and fork-tender.
5. Transfer the potatoes to a serving platter, squeeze the fresh lemon juice over them, and sprinkle with parsley. Serve hot.

Fresh Green Beans with Bacon, Mushrooms & Herbs

Prep Time: 15 minutes // Cook Time: 20 minutes

Thanksgiving | Christmas | New Year

Servings: 6 Servings

Course: Side Dishes

Calories: 94kcal

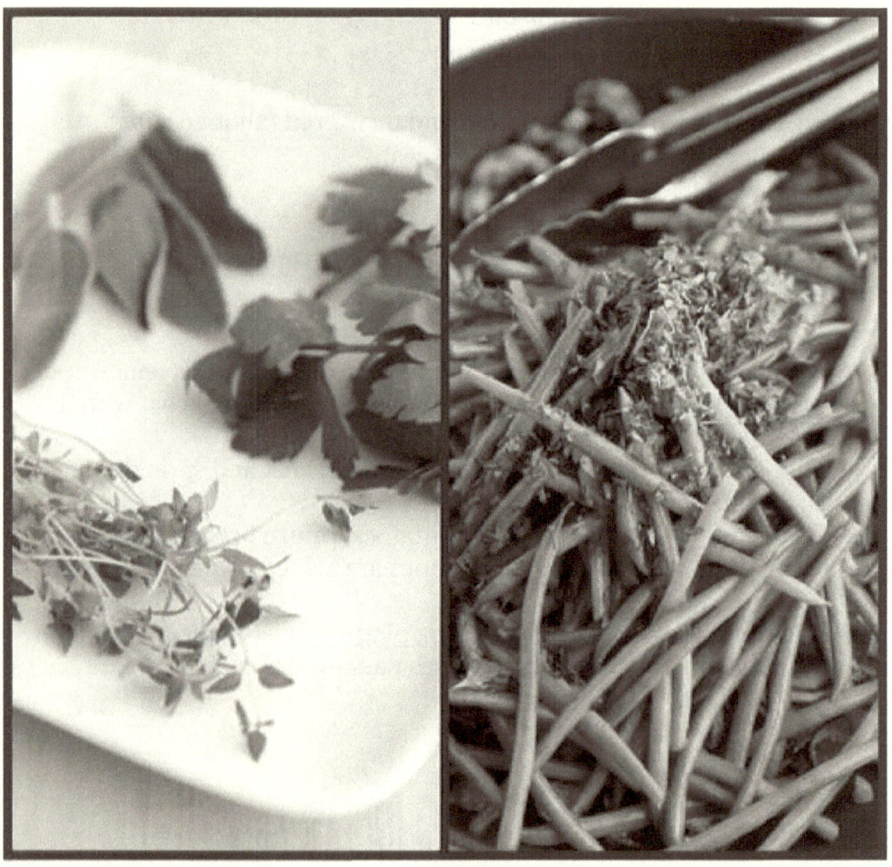

Fresh green beans are tossed with crispy bacon, sautéed mushrooms, shallots and fresh herbs. This is a wonderful, bright side for your Thanksgiving feast.

Ingredients

- 1 pound thin green beans trimmed

* 3 strips bacon
* 1 large shallot minced
* 12 ounces mushrooms thinly sliced
* 1 teaspoon olive oil
* 3 tablespoons parsley minced
* 1 tablespoon minced fresh thyme leaves
* 1 tablespoon minced fresh sage
* 1/4 teaspoon kosher salt
* 1/4 teaspoon freshly ground black pepper

Instructions

1. Bring a large saucepan of salted water to a boil. Add the beans and cook until tender-crisp, about 2 minutes. Drain and immediately transfer the beans to a bowl of ice water to stop the cooking.
2. Drain the beans again and set aside.
3. Place the strips of bacon in a large skillet set over medium heat. Cook until the bacon is crisp. Transfer to a paper towel, then crumble the bacon and set aside.
4. Discard all but 1 teaspoon of the bacon fat. Add the olive oil to the bacon fat in the skillet, and turn to medium-high heat. Add the shallots and mushrooms, and cook until tender, 2 to 3 minutes.
5. Add the green beans and cook for 1 to 2 minutes, stirring frequently.
6. Add the parsley, thyme, sage, salt and pepper, and stir to combine. Cook for an additional minute, then add the bacon.
7. Serve hot or at room temperature.

Nutrition

Serving: 1Serving (1/6 of Recipe) | Calories: 94kcal | Carbohydrates: 9g | Protein: 5g | Fat: 5g | Saturated Fat: 2g | Cholesterol: 7mg | Sodium: 179mg | Potassium: 394mg | Fiber: 3g | Sugar: 4g | Vitamin A: 745IU | Vitamin C: 15.3mg | Calcium: 44mg | Iron: 1.6mg

Roasted Potato

Prep Time: 15 minutes // Cook Time: 20 minutes

Thanksgiving | Christmas | New Year | Easter | Halloween

Servings: 8 Servings

Course: Side Dishes

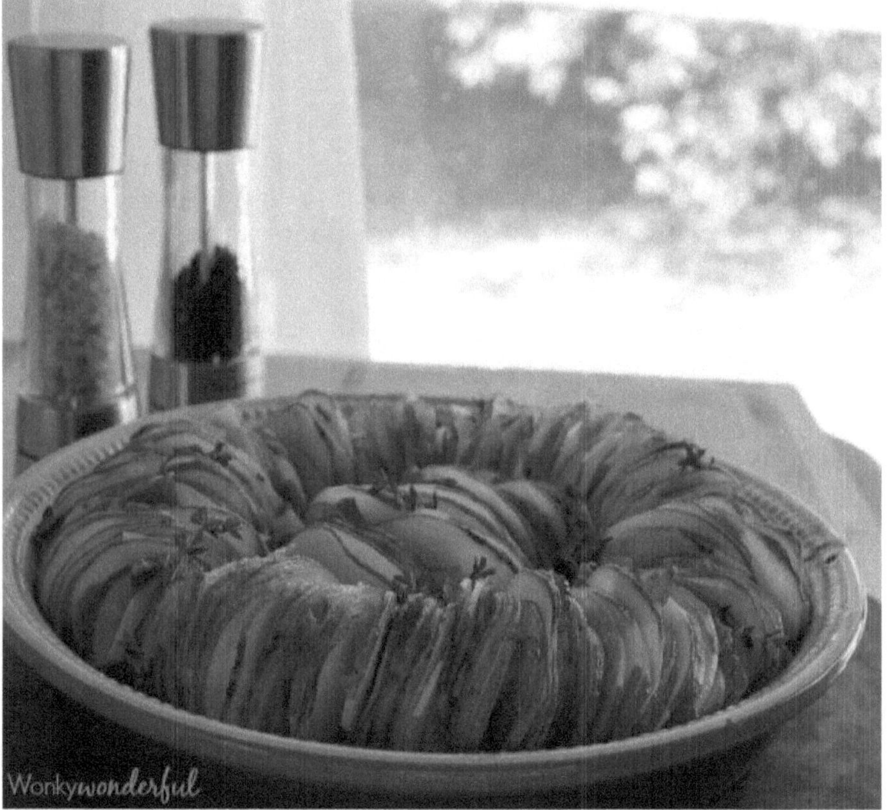

Ingredients

- lbs Red Potatoes
- 5-6 Strips Soft Cooked Bacon - cut into pieces
- Tablespoons Olive Oil*
- 2 teaspoons Fresh Lemon Juice
- 10 Cloves Roasted Garlic - smashed into a paste
- 1-2 Tablespoons Olive Oil, additional
- 3 Sprigs Thyme
- Fresh Cracked Himalayan Salt and Black Pepper

Instructions

1   Preheat oven to 375°
2   Mix 5 Tb olive oil, lemon juice and roasted garlic paste in a large bowl. Thoroughly clean potatoes.
3   Thinly slice potatoes with mandoline. (approximately 1/8 inch) Toss potatoes in olive oil mixture until evenly coated. Arrange potato slices (accordion style) in a 10 inch pie plate. Bake for 1 hour.
4   Remove from oven. Brush 1-2 Tb olive oil over the tops of potato slices. Tuck bacon pieces and thyme between potato slices. Generously salt and pepper with the Cole & Mason Mills. Return to oven and bake 30-35 minutes or until potatoes are cooked through. Potatoes should be soft in the middle and crisp on the outer edges.
5   Serve with additional salt and pepper to taste.

Notes

*I used some of the oil left over from roasted garlic.

Oven Roasted Carrots

Prep time: 5 Mins // Cook time: 25 Mins

Yield: 4

Thanksgiving | Christmas | New Year | Easter | Halloween

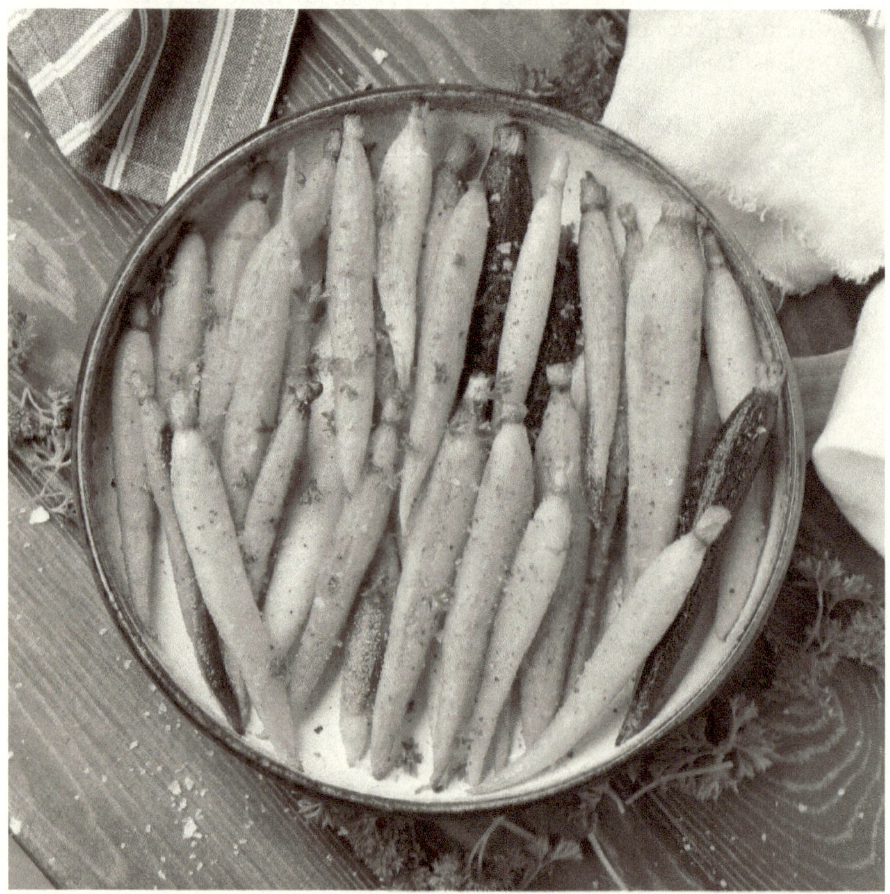

Save some time and make an easy holiday side dish. These Oven Roasted Carrots are a super simple side for your holiday menu or with a weeknight dinner. Rainbow carrots spiced with Adobo seasoning and roasted in the oven. This is a Whole foods compliant Paleo recipe, vegan and vegetarian.

Ingredients

- 2 Lbs Rainbow Carrots, (trimmed, washed)
- 2 Tablespoons Olive Oil
- 1 teaspoon Adobo Seasoning

Instructions

1. Preheat oven to 400°F
2. Toss carrots with olive oil and seasoning. Transfer to a lightly oiled rimmed baking sheet. Make sure the baking sheet is large enough that the carrots are spread out, otherwise use 2 baking sheets.
3. Roast carrots for 15 minutes.
4. Rotate carrots, increase temp to 425°F and roast for 10-15 more minutes or until tender and golden brown.
5. Sprinkle with salt, pepper, fresh parsley and serve.

Chive horseradish cauliflower mash

Prep Time: 10 minutes // Cook Time: 25 minutes

Thanksgiving | Christmas | New Year | Easter | Halloween

Makes 8 servings – 3 grams of net carbs per serving

Category: Side Dishes

Yield: 8 servings

Method: Steaming

This Chive Horseradish Keto Cauliflower Mash is the last potato substitution recipe you will ever need. Rich, flavorful, and utterly delicious

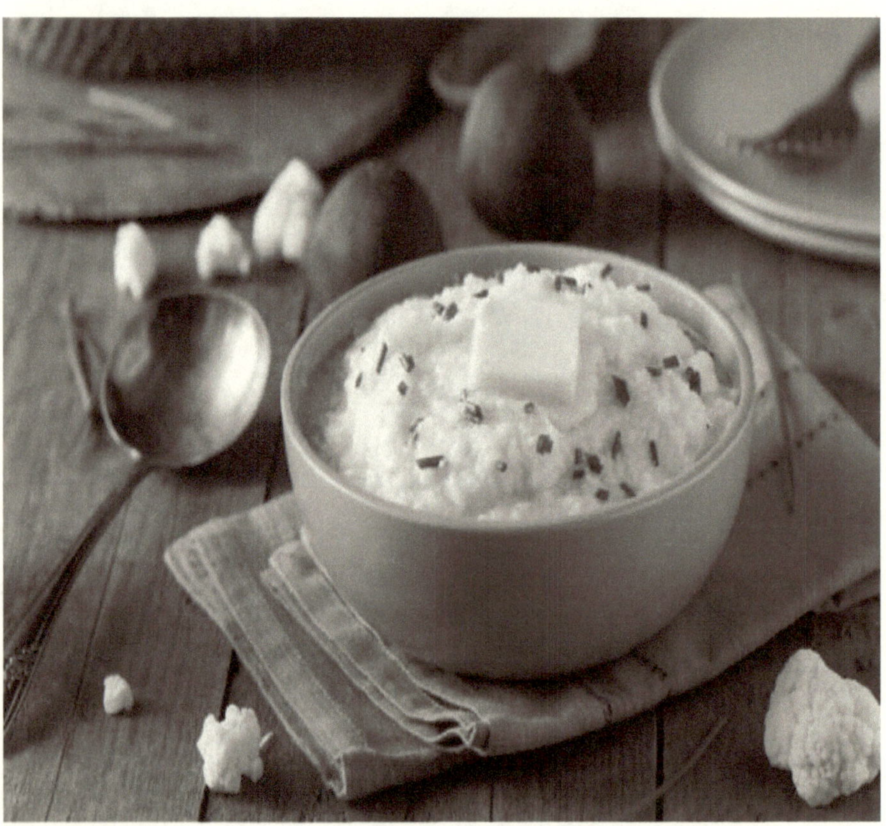

Ingredients

- 1 large head of cauliflower

- 5 chives, chopped, extra for garnish
- 1/2 cup grated Parmesan cheese
- 3 tablespoons coconut oil, extra for garnish
- 3 tablespoons creamy horseradish sauce, or 1 1/2 tablespoons prepared horseradish
- 1/2 cup sour cream
- 3 cloves garlic, minced
- sea salt and ground black pepper, to taste

Instructions

1. Over medium-high heat, steam cauliflower in a covered pot in 1 to 2 inches of water. Steam until the cauliflower is fork tender, about 15 minutes.
2. Turn off the burner, drain the water and leave the cauliflower in the hot pot. This will help pull some of the excess moisture from the cauliflower. This step is crucial to not having soupy cauliflower mash.
3. Once the excess liquid is gone and the cauliflower feels fairly dry, fork mash the cauliflower.
4. Add the chives, Parmesan cheese, coconut oil, horseradish, sour cream, garlic, salt and pepper. Mash until all ingredients are well incorporated and the cauliflower is the consistency of mashed potatoes.
5. Garnish with extra chives and coconut oil before serving.

Bacon Wrapped Brussels Sprouts with Balsamic Mayo Dip

Prep Time 10 minutes // Cook Time 40 minutes

Thanksgiving | Christmas | New Year | Easter | Halloween

Servings 4 servings

Calories 170 kcal

A favorite fall appetizer -- roasted brussels sprouts wrapped with crispy bacon slices, dipped in a balsamic vinegar and mayonnaise sauce.

Fall, gluten free, oven, paleo, Thanksgiving, whole, winter

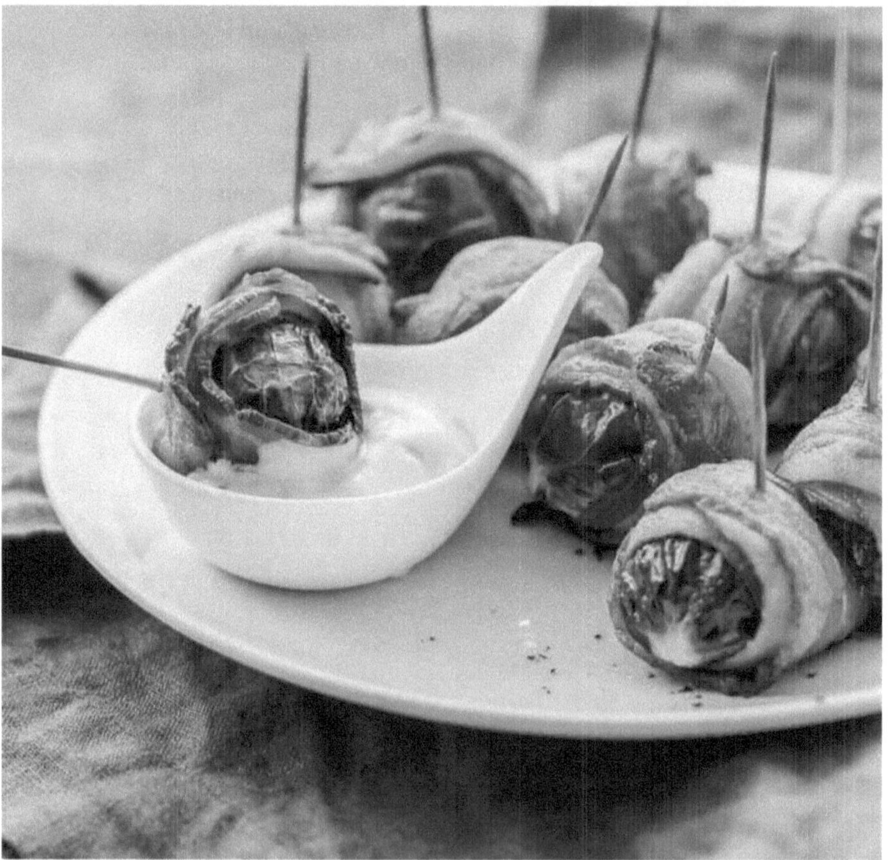

Ingredients

- 12 slices bacon

- 12 brussels sprouts (about 12 ounces) stems trimmed
- 12 toothpicks
- For the balsamic dip:
- 5 tablespoons mayonnaise
- 1 tablespoon balsamic vinegar

Instructions

1. Prepare a baking tray lined with parchment paper or a baking mat.
2. Preheat the oven to 400 F.
3. Wrap a bacon slice around each brussels sprout, and secure with a toothpick. Place in a single layer on the baking tray.
4. Bake at 400 F until the bacon is crispy and the brussels sprouts are very tender, about 40 minutes.
5. Combine mayonnaise and balsamic vinegar together in a small bowl. Stir until smooth.
6. Serve the bacon wrapped brussels sprouts with the balsamic mayonnaise dip.

Nutrition Info

This recipe yields 2.5 g net carbs per serving.

Calories 170, Total Fat 15g 24%, Saturated Fat 1g 6%, Trans Fat 0g, Cholesterol 13mg 4%, Sodium 120mg 5%, Potassium 0mg 0%, Total Carb 5g 2%, Dietary Fiber 2.5g 9%, Sugars 2g, Protein 2g, Vitamin A 6% · Vitamin C 90% · Calcium 2% · Iron 0%

Umami Gravy

This gravy is pure, unadulterated umami. I recommend freezing some in an ice cube tray so you'll always have individual servings of gravy at the ready. Perfect for your Whole Thanksgiving!

Ingredients

- ½ ounce dried porcini mushrooms
- 2 tablespoons ghee or fat of choice
- 2 onions diced
- 1 teaspoon tomato paste
- ½ teaspoon fish sauce
- ½ pound cremini mushrooms sliced
- 3 garlic cloves minced
- 4 cups bone broth or organic chicken stock
- 3 fresh thyme sprigs
- kosher salt
- freshly ground black pepper

Instructions

1. Rinse the dried mushrooms with cool water and place them in a small bowl. Add enough water to cover the mushrooms and set aside for at least 30 minutes to soften.
2. In a medium saucepan, melt the ghee over medium heat. Add in the onions and sauté for 10 to 15 minutes or until translucent.
3. Then, drop in the tomato paste and fish sauce. Stir to evenly distribute the umami boosters, before dumping in the sliced cremini mushrooms. Cook the mushrooms until the liquid is released and evaporated, about 10 minutes.
4. In the meantime, fish the reconstituted porcini mushrooms out of the bowl of water, and roughly chop them up.
5. Add the garlic to the saucepan, and cook for 30 seconds or until fragrant.
6. Then, mix in the reconstituted dried mushrooms, pour in the broth, and drop in the thyme sprigs. Increase the heat to high and bring the gravy to a boil.

7. Decrease heat to medium-low to maintain a strong simmer/low boil, and cook until the gravy has reduced by half, about 30 minutes. Be patient—you want half of the liquid to evaporate in order to concentrate the flavors. Plus, you don't want the gravy to be thin and watery once blended.

8. Remove from the heat. Take out the thyme twigs and season to taste with salt and pepper.

9. Using an immersion blender or a regular blender, purée the gravy until smooth.

Notes

Don't worry—the smidge of fish sauce doesn't make your gravy fishy; it just amps up the umami.

Dijon Pomegranate Salmon

Prep: 20 minutes | Cook Time: 8 minutes

Thanksgiving | Christmas | Birthday

Serves 4

This recipe is ridiculously easy to make yet elegant, delicious and beautiful! Add some green herbs for a red and green theme! Perfect for holiday brunch or party of any spread for versatility!

Ingredients:

- 1.5lb side (whole filet) of wild caught salmon
- 1 teaspoon fine salt
- 1 teaspoon onion powder
- 1 tablespoons Dijon mustard
- 2 tablespoons coconut aminos
- 2 tablespoons avocado oil
- ½ cup pomegranate arils

Instructions

1. Lay your salmon on a parchment paper lined sheet pan and sprinkle with salt.
2. In a small bowl mix the onion powder, Dijon, coconut aminos and avocado oil
3. Spread this mix all over the salmon and let it rest for 10-15 minutes at room temperature before cooking.
4. Set to cook on the top rack of your oven at 550F. Cookfor7-8 minutes or until thickest part of the salmon easily flakes. Remove from the oven, transfer to your serving platter or tray, spoon the pomegranate arils over the salmon.
5. You may also add fresh dill or parsley

Dijon Pomegranate Roasted Brussel Sprouts

(Paleo + Keto Thanksgiving Menu)

Prep Time: 5 mins Cook Time: 30 mins

Thanksgiving | Christmas | New Year

Ingredients

- 1 pound Brussel sprouts, halved
- 4 cloves garlic, sliced
- ½ teaspoon salt
- 4 tablespoons coconut oil
- 2 tablespoon coconut aminos
- 2 tablespoons Dijon mustard
- 2 tablespoon coconut or red wine vinegar
- 1 teaspoon ground ginger
- 3 tablespoons pomegranate seeds

Instructions

1. Pre-heat the oven to 400F. Place the Brussel sprouts and sliced garlic on the sheet pan. Sprinkle with salt.
2. In a small bowl melt the fat then mix in the coconut aminos, mustard, vinegar and pomegranate seeds.
3. Pour half of the sauce over the veggies and toss to combine. Save the rest for after.
4. Then spread the brussel sprouts out over the sheet pan.
5. Roast for 30 minutes or until crispy.
6. Use a thin spatula to scrape all the goodness off of the sheet pan. Mix and serve.
7. Drizzle the remaining sauce over the Brussel sprouts.
8. Garnish with a few extra pomegranate seeds!

Recipe Notes:

If cooking more than a pound at a time, and if the sheet pan is a little more crowded you shoukd use two sheet pans and increase the cooking time by 5 minutes as needed.

Low Carb Sugar-Free Cranberry Sauce Recipe – 4 Ingredients

Cook Time 10 minutes // Total Time 10 minutes

Servings: 6 servings (1/4 cup each)

Thanksgiving | Christmas | New Year | Easter | Halloween

Course Appetizer, Side Dish

Calories 32 kcal

This healthy, sugar-free cranberry sauce recipe requires just 4 ingredients. Made with fresh cranberries and no sugar, it's also low carb, paleo, and gluten-free.

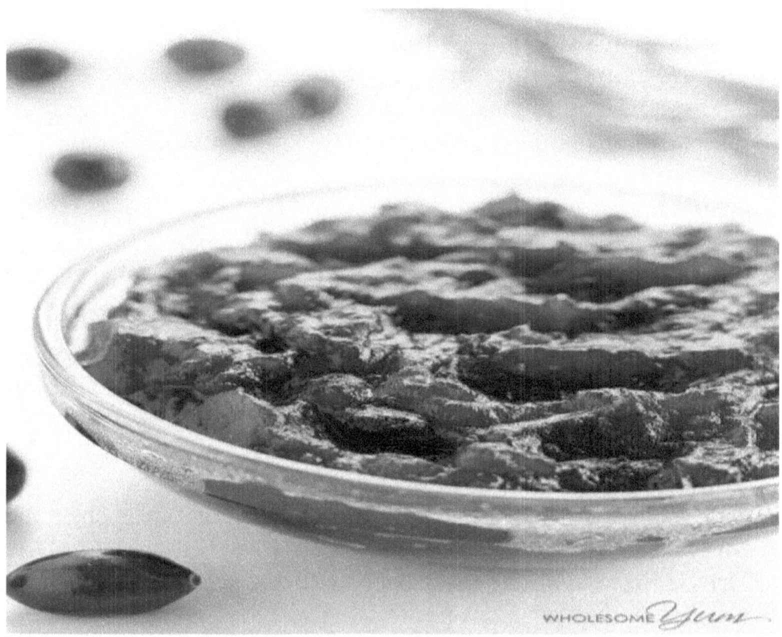

Ingredients

- 12 oz Cranberries
- 1 cup Powdered erythritol *See notes
- 3/4 cup Water
- 1 tsp Orange zest (optional; add more if you like more orange flavor)
- 1/2 tsp Vanilla extract

Instructions

1. Combine the cranberries, water, erythritol, and orange zest in a medium saucepan. Bring to a boil, then reduce heat to a gentle simmer.
2. Simmer for 10-15 minutes, until the cranberries pop and a sauce forms.
3. Remove from heat. Stir in the vanilla extract.

RECIPE NOTES

If you want your sugar-free cranberry sauce to keep for longer without crystallizing, use powdered erythritol. If you'll be using it right away, regular granulated erythritol (or any granulated sweetener) will work just fine.

Calories32, Fat0g, Protein0g, Total Carbs6g, Net Carbs4g, Fiber2g, Sugar2g

Bacon-wrapped maple Parmesan Asparagus bundles

Prep Time: 15 minutes // Cook Time: 40 minutes

Thanksgiving | Christmas | New Year

Yield: 8 bundles

Category: Appetizer

Method: Bake

These Bacon-Wrapped Maple Parmesan Asparagus Bundles are a delicious low-carb and keto-friendly party appetizer

This recipe is **keto, low-carb, nut-free, egg-free, coconut-free, gluten-free, grain-free, refined-sugar-free, and contains only 2.9 grams of net carbs per serving!**

Ingredients

- 1/2 cup maple-flavored syrup (use code "REALBALANCED" for 20% off Lakanto products)
- 1/2 cup unsalted coconut oil
- 1/2 tsp salt
- 1/4 tsp black pepper
- 2 lbs fresh asparagus, washed, ends chopped off
- 8 slices thick-cut bacon
- 20g (2 tbsp + 2 tsp) grated parmesan

Instructions

1. Preheat oven to 425 degrees.
2. To a small pot over medium low heat, add maple-flavored syrup, coconut oil, salt, and pepper and bring to a light boil, whisking occasionally. Remove from heat and set aside.
3. Split asparagus stalks into 8 groups. Wrap bacon slices around grouped asparagus stalks, starting about 1/2 inch from the bottom, and secure bacon slice with toothpick. Transfer bacon-wrapped asparagus bundles to casserole dish.
4. Pour syrup mixture into casserole dish atop bundled asparagus and sprinkle half of grated parmesan (~10g) on top. Bake for 35-40 minutes.
5. While asparagus bundles cook in oven, place baking rack atop a foil-lined line baking sheet.
6. Remove casserole dish from oven and transfer baked bundles to prepared baking rack (rotating them so the side that was baked

down is now up), turn on oven broiler, and broil until bacon is crispy, about 1-2 minutes.

7. Remove baking sheet from oven, remove toothpicks from bundles, sprinkle remaining grated parmesan on top, and allow to cool slightly prior to serving.

Lemony Prosciutto-Wrapped Asparagus

Prep Time: 10 Mins // Cook Time: 15 Mins

Thanksgiving | Christmas | New Year | Easter | Halloween

Yield: 4

Recipe Type: Side Dish

A quick and easy side dish or appetizer that is Whole, paleo, and Keto friendly!

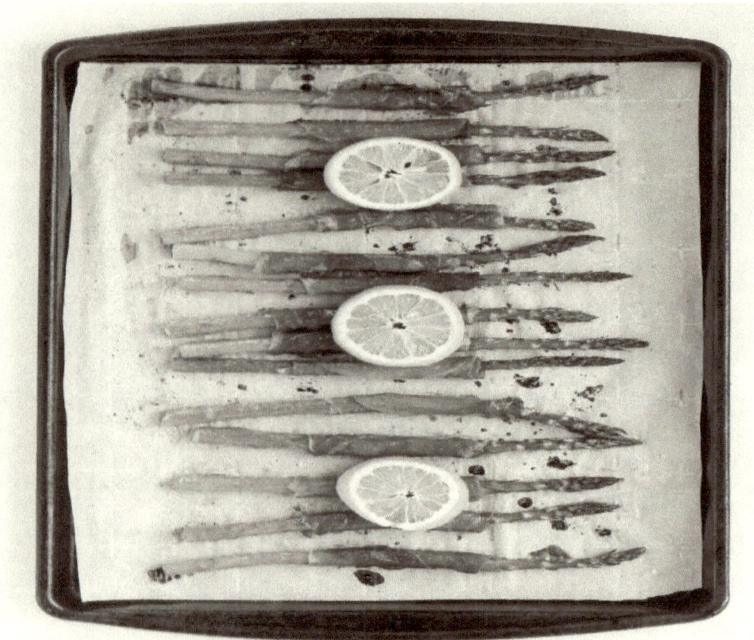

Ingredients

- 16 pieces asparagus ends trimmed
- 8 pieces prosciutto
- 1 lemon
- olive oil or avocado oil spray

Instructions

1. Preheat oven to 450. Line a baking sheet with foil or parchment paper.

2.   Cut all of the prosciutto pieces in half. Wrap one half around each piece of asparagus, tucking the ends underneath to hold in place.
3.   Place the wrapped asparagus pieces on the baking sheet, making sure to leave some room in between each piece.
4.   Spray the pieces of asparagus with oil (lightly). Cut your lemon in half, and squeeze one half over all of the asparagus.
5.   Slice the other half into rounds and place them on top of the asparagus. Bake for 12 mins. Enjoy!

Low Carb Cucumber Salad (Thai)

Prep Time 15 minutes

Thanksgiving | Christmas | New Year | Easter | Halloween

Servings 4 people

Calories 75kcal

An easy and refreshing Thai cucumber salad that takes mere minutes to prepare. This low carb recipe is sugar-free and perfect for any ketogenic diet.

Ingredients

- 16 ounces English cucumber peeled (about 1 large cucumber)
- 1/4 cup chopped cilantro
- 2-3 scallions, thinly sliced

Dressing

- 1/4 cup white vinegar
- 1/4 cup Sukrin Melis (Sukrin Icing Sugar or Swerve Confectioners) or your favorite sweetener to taste
- 1 tablespoon Red Boat Fish Sauce, or your favorite
- 1 tablespoon water
- 1 teaspoon toasted sesame oil
- 1/2 teaspoon salt
- 1 ounce crushed peanuts or 1 tablespoon sesame seeds

Optional Toppings

- Thai red chiles thinly sliced
- carrots thinly sliced or grated
- purple cabbage thinly sliced for color

Instructions

Preparation:

1. Peel the cucumber and spiralize into noodles or slice and cut into 1/2 rounds or quarters.
2. Slice the scallion, chop the cilantro, and slice any of the additional toppings if using. Cover and refrigerate until needed.

Dressing:

1. Add all of the ingredients for the dressing to a small bowl and stir to dissolve the sweetener. Taste. It should be sweet, sour, and salty and balanced to your taste buds.
2. Cover and refrigerate until needed.

Mix:

1. Assemble the salad just a few minutes before serving by tossing the ingredients with the dressing.

Amount Per Serving

Calories: 75kcal | Carbohydrates: 6g | Protein: 5g | Fat: 5g | Fiber: 2g

Low Carb Pizza Chicken Skillet

Prep Time 5 minutes // Cook Time 15 minutes

Thanksgiving | Christmas | New Year | Easter | Halloween

Servings 5 people

Calories 337kcal

An easy low carb chicken skillet recipe that's so simple to prepare. Just brown boneless skinless chicken meat and smother with pizza toppings.

Ingredients

- 2 tablespoons avocado oil or olive oil
- 1.5 pounds skinless/boneless chicken pieces about 5 thighs
- 1/4 teaspoon salt sprinkle to taste
- 1/8 teaspoon pepper sprinkle to taste
- 2 cloves garlic minced
- 1 cup low carb pizza sauce or marinara sauce
- 5 slices mozzarellaVegan cheese
- 1 ounce pepperoni slices

Instructions

1. Heat oil in skillet over medium high heat. Season chicken with salt and pepper.
2. Add seasoned chicken and garlic to skillet. Cook chicken until browned.
3. Pour pizza or marinara sauce on top. Allow to simmer until sauce is heated.
4. Top each piece of chicken with a slice of mozzarella cheese and pieces of pepperoni.
5. Cover skillet until cheese is melted or place skillet under broiler to melt cheese. Serve immediately.

Amount Per Serving (1 piece)

Calories 337 Calories from Fat 162

Net Carbs 2g, Carbs: 2.5%, Protein: 46.5%, Fat: 50.9%

Total Fat 18g 28%, Saturated Fat 5g 25%, Polyunsaturated Fat 1g, Total Carbohydrates 3g 1%, Dietary Fiber 1g 4%, Sugars 1g, Protein 37g 74%, Vitamin A 5%, Vitamin C 0%, Calcium 14%, Iron 3%

Harvest Vegetable Hash

Prep time: 5mins // Cook time: 60 mins

Thanksgiving | Christmas

Yield: 4-5 Serving

Course: Side

Paleo, Whole, Aip

Ingredients

- 2 slices of bacon
- 1 large sweet potato, chopped
- 2 medium carrots, chopped
- 1 medium rutabaga, chopped
- 2 cups brussels sprouts, halved
- 1 medium yellow onion, diced
- 2 tsp sage
- 2 tsp rosemary (plus more for garnish)
- 2 tsp thyme
- 1/2 tsp sea salt

Instructions

1. Preheat the oven to 400 F and line a baking sheet with parchment paper.
2. Place the bacon slices on the baking sheet and bake in the oven for 18-20 minutes, or until the bacon is just cooked. Be sure not to over crisp it as it will be re-crisped in the oven. Chop the bacon and set it aside. Reserve the fat in the pan.
3. Add all of the vegetables to the baking sheet with the herbs and salt and toss in the baking fat to evenly coat.
4. Bake the vegetables in the oven for 30-40 minutes, or until crisp. Cook time will vary depending on sizes. Add the chopped bacon to the vegetable mix for the final 2-3 minutes to re-crisp and heat.
5. Remove the vegetable hash from the oven and top with additional herbs for garnish and salt to taste.

Serving size: 1 serving

Calories: 125, fat: 4.8g, carbohydrates: 18.1g, fiber: 4.8g, protein: 4.2g

Roasted Sweet Potatoes with Cauliflower Cream Sauce

Prep Time: 20 mins // Cook Time: 50 mins

Thanksgiving | Christmas

Course: Side Dish

Servings: 5 Servings

Calories: 175 kcal

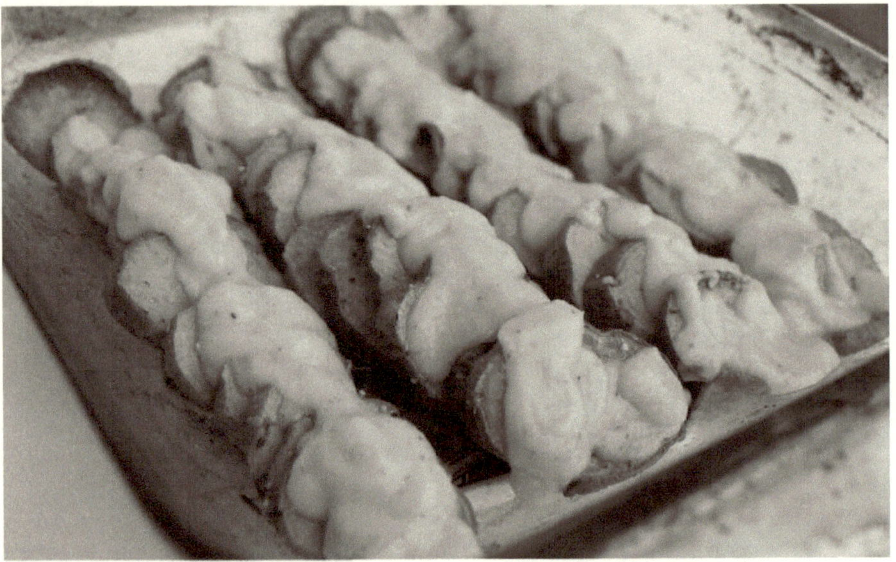

These roasted sweet potatoes with cauliflower cream sauce would make a great side for any old weeknight dinner or even for a holiday dinner like thanksgiving or christmas!

Ingredients

For the sweet potatoes:
- 3 medium sweet potatoes
- 2 tbsp extra virgin olive oil
- 1 tsp sea salt
- 1/2 tsp black pepper (omit for AIP)
- 1/2 tsp thyme
- 1/2 tsp oregano

For the cauliflower sauce:
- 1 medium cauliflower

- 3/4 cup bone broth (or vegetable broth for vegan)
- 2 cloves garlic
- 1/2 tsp sea salt
- 1/2 tsp black pepper (omit for AIP)
- 1/2 tsp sage
- 1/2 tsp thyme
- 1/2 tsp onion powder
- 1 tbsp olive oil

Instructions

For the sweet potatoes:

1. First, preheat the oven to 400°.
2. Wash the sweet potatoes, then slice them into thin slices about 1/2 inch wide. Place them in a bowl and drizzle with the olive oil and sprinkle with the salt, pepper and spices.
3. Stir the sweet potatoes around in the bowl to coat each slice with olive oil and spices.
4. Place them stacked in a slanted direction in rows across a 8x8 pyrex baking dish. Bake for about 45-55 minutes.

For the cauliflower sauce:

1. First, wash the cauliflower heads and chop them into small pieces. Place the chopped cauliflower into a large pot and pour in the broth.
2. The broth should come up just short of the top of the cauliflower, it shouldn't be covering the cauliflower. Add more if necessary. Turn on the heat to high.
3. Add in the whole garlic cloves (they do not need to be chopped since they will be pureed later). Then add in the salt, pepper, spices and stir. Cover the pot with a lid and bring it to a boil.
4. Once the cauliflower is boiling, stir it and turn the heat to medium-high (it should continue to boil gently).
5. Let it cook for about 30 minutes or until the cauliflower is very soft and tender. You should be able to easily mash it with a fork. Turn the heat off.
6. If you are using a hand blender you can immediately begin to puree the cauliflower until it is smooth, but be careful not to let it splash since it's hot.
7. If you are using a blender to puree it, wait for it to cool, but first add the olive oil. Then, once it's cooled blend it until it becomes a smooth puree.
8. If you used a hand blender, add the coconut oil or olive oil after you've pureed it and then puree it once more to blend the oil.
9. Pour your desired amount of cauliflower puree over the roasted potatoes and enjoy!

Calories 175Calories from Fat 72, Fat 8g12%, Saturated Fat 2g13%, Cholesterol 6mg2%, Sodium 810mg35%, Potassium 614mg18%, Carbohydrates 22g7%, Fiber 4g17%, Sugar 5g6%, Protein 4g8%, Vitamin A 11135IU223%, Vitamin C 58.9mg71%, Calcium 51mg5%, Iron 1mg6%

Brazilian Garlicky Collard Greens (Couve a Mineira)

Prep time: 5 minutes//Cook time: 10 minutes

Thanksgiving | Christmas

Course: Side Dish

Servings: 2 Servings

Ingredients

- 1 bunch collard greens
- 4-6 cloves garlic
- 1/4 tsp sea salt
- 2 Tbsp extra virgin olive oil (or coconut oil)

Instructions

1. Rinse and pat dry collard leaves.
2. Cut out tough center stem with a knife in a V shape as pictured, then continue to cut leaf in half.
3. Stack about 6 leaf halves together and roll them up tightly.
4. Cut crosswise strips about a quarter inch wide. Try to keep the strips together and in place.
5. Next, cut the thin strips in half with one long lengthwise cut down the middle.
6. Repeat steps 2-5 until all leaves are cut into strips.
7. For traditional preparation, use a mortar and pestle to mash garlic with salt. You can also use a press on the garlic or finely mince with your knife and mix with salt.
8. Heat olive oil in pan over medium-low heat for about 1 minute.
9. Add garlic and salt and saute until garlic is fragrant, about 1-2 minutes.
10. Add collard strips and saute, stirring frequently, until they are softened and bright green in color. They will reduce in volume by about half (sometimes more).
11. Watch them carefully to avoid overcooking. You do not want them to start turning dark.
12. Total cooking time with vary depending on your stove and cookware, but should take between about 4-8 minutes.
13. Serve immediately and enjoy!

Paleo & AIP Pear Upside Down Cake with Easy Caramel Sauce

Prep Time: 25 mins//Cook Time: 30 mins

New Year | Easter | Halloween

Servings: 8 servings

Upside down cakes are the epitome of pleasurable desserts: moistest of cakes, caramelized fruit and the option of whipped cream.

This beautiful fall dessert is egg-free and dairy-free, and you'll love making and using the caramel sauce — just three ingredients and five minutes of cooking.

Enjoy making a beautiful Paleo and AIP dessert for yourself and the ones you love.

Ingredients

- 2 whole pears peeled
- 1 cup unsweetened applesauce
- 2/3 cup filtered water
- 2/3 cup coconut butter warmed slightly
- 1/2 cup cassava flour
- 1/3 cup coconut flour
- 1/4 cup fat of choice melted and cooled slightly, if solid fat
- 1/4 cup coconut sugar
- 1 Tablespoon apple cider vinegar
- 1 Tablespoon gelatin, see Recipe Notes for discount code and link
- 1/2 teaspoon baking soda, sifted
- 1/4 teaspoon dried ginger
- 1/4 teaspoon cinnamon
- 1/4 teaspoon sea salt

Easy AIP Caramel Sauce

- 1/3 cup coconut cream
- 1/4 cup coconut sugar
- pinch sea salt

Instructions

1. Place coconut cream and coconut sugar in small saucepan. Turn heat to medium and bring to simmer, stirring to dissolve sugar.

2   Once simmering, reduce heat to very low and maintain simmer for 5 minutes. Stir occasionally. Turn off heat and stir in sea salt. Set aside.
3   Preheat oven to 350 degrees.
4   Grease 9" round cake pan. Slice pears and arrange decoratively around the base of the cake pan. (This will become the top of the cake.)
5   In large bowl stir together wet cake ingredients and sugar: applesauce, warm coconut butter, warm water, fat, apple cider vinegar and coconut sugar.
6   In smaller bowl sift together dry ingredients: cassava flour, coconut flour, gelatin, baking soda, ginger, cinnamon and sea salt.
7   Pour dry ingredients into wet ingredients and fold together until well mixed, without over-mixing.
8   Pour caramel sauce somewhat evenly over pears in cake pan. (Don't worry about spreading it evenly.) Scoop out batter and spread it evenly over the caramel and pears in the pan.
9   Bake in preheated oven 30 minutes. Remove to cooling rack for 10 minutes.
10 We unmold the cake while it's still warm so the caramel top and pears come away from the pan easily.)
11 Carefully flip cake over onto plate or serving platter. (Do this by placing plate on top of pan.
12 Hold both pan and plate together tightly and quickly flip.)
13 Lift off cake pan. If any pears are displaced, simply put them back into place. Allow cake to cool completely.
14 Serve alone or embellish with coconut whipped cream.

Sweet Potato and Broccoli Soup

Allergen friendly, dairy free, AIP, paleo & Whole friendly!

Christmas | New Year | Easter | Halloween

Yield: 4

Ingredients

- 3/4 lb / 340 g white sweet potato
- 1/2 lb / 225 g broccoli florets
- 1 leek
- 1 medium onion
- 4 cups / 960 ml chicken broth
- 2 tsp / 2 g dried oregano leaves
- 1 tsp / 5g fine sea salt
- 1 2/3 cup / 400 ml full fat coconut milk

To garnish:

- Drizzle of lemon olive oil
- Chopped green onion tops
- Chopped fresh chives

Instructions

1. Peel and chop the white sweet potato into evenly sized chunks. Chop any large broccoli florets in half so that all the pieces are about the same size as the sweet potato pieces.
2. Cut the leek in half through the root and carefully rinse out any dirt or grit from between the layers under cold running water, then slice the leek into half moons about a 1/2 inch thick.
3. Peel and dice the onion. Add all the chopped vegetables to a saucepan or dutch oven large enough to have at least an inch of head room at the top.

SIMMER:

1. Pour the chicken broth over the vegetables and add the dried oregano and salt.
2. Bring the liquid to a steady simmer and continue to cook until the vegetables are tender, about 25 minutes.

BLEND:

1. Remove the pan from the heat and add the coconut milk (I like to add it at the end like this so that it doesn't have a chance to

accidentally overheat and separate, plus I find I get a creamier texture this way).

2   Use an immersion blender to carefully puree the soup together until smooth, then taste and add any additional seasonings if you wish.

3   Garnish just before serving with a drizzle of lemon olive oil and some chopped green onion tops and fresh chives.

4   I like to make a double batch of this soup at the weekend and then eat it throughout the week for breakfast: it will easily last a week in the fridge.

INDEX